METHOD
MEETS ART

Arts-Based Research Practice

Patricia Leavy

THE GUILFORD PRESS
New York   London

© 2009 The Guilford Press
A Division of Guilford Publications, Inc.
72 Spring Street, New York, NY 10012
www.guilford.com

Printed in the United States of America

This book is printed on acid-free paper.

Last digit is print number: 9   8   7   6   5   4   3   2

Library of Congress Cataloging-in-Publication Data

Leavy, Patricia, 1975–
   Method meets art : arts-based research practice / by Patricia Leavy.
     p. cm.
   Includes bibliographical references and index.
   ISBN 978-1-59385-843-8 (hbk.)—ISBN 978-1-59385-259-7 (pbk.)
    1. Qualitative research—Methodology. 2. Art and society. 3. Art and science.
I. Title.
   H62.L395 2009
   700.72—dc22

                              2008012632

*To my mother, Sylvia,
and my daughter, Madeline*

Preface

When I entered the graduate program in sociology at Boston College, I was fortunate to end up in a required research methods course taught, at the time, by Sharlene Hesse-Biber. Sharlene is a feminist scholar and qualitative methodologist. As a result of her *holistic approach* to the research process—which emphasizes the interconnections between epistemology, theory, and methods—I too developed a holistic understanding of social research congruent with my long-term social justice commitments.

As graduate school was nearing completion and I was entering the world of "publish or perish" and scant funding opportunities, I soon realized that the disciplinary research demands experienced by those in many academic disciplines called for a far more limited view of research than I had hoped. For instance, research published in top-tier sociology journals was largely quantitative and relied on the replication of research procedures and the like. Published qualitative research often followed strict disciplinary standards regarding methodological choices, at times seemingly judged against inappropriate positivist standards. Moreover, discussions of theory often appeared separate from discussions of method, failing to provide holistic accounts of the research endeavor. Innovative qualitative methods, such as autoethnography and ethnodrama, seemed to be relegated to a lower or "experimental" status, thereby undercutting the effectiveness of the research.

Like so many others who want to show their folks that they have "done something with their lives," I proudly gave my father copies of my first few publications. Although highly educated himself, he responded that he was proud of me but unable to read my work—it "looks impressive but there is too much jargon, I just don't get it," he said. Frankly, I didn't get it either. I didn't get what I was spending all of my time on. The research tools I was using were inadequate for accessing the often invisible and intangible aspects of social life, such as the multi-tude of subtle effects of ideological systems in daily life and the range of complex feelings underlying research participants' attitudes and experiences, that I as a lifelong feminist was after. What's worse, it almost didn't matter because such a small circle of people would ever even have the possibility of reading my work. And the work had officially started *feeling like work.* Joyless. I wasn't expressing what I wanted to, to whom I wanted. I needed to find a *different way* to conduct research.

It was at this point that I again worked with my methods mentor, Sharlene, on two projects about "emergent methods," our term for innovative approaches to research. It was during this period that I began to discover the world of arts-based research (ABR) practices through the pioneering work of Mary Beth Cancienne, Elliot Eisner, Carolyn Ellis, Rita Irwin, Kip Jones, Ronald Pelias, Johnny Saldaña, and Celeste Snowber, to name just a few. I began adapting these approaches to my own empirical projects in the areas of collective memory, body image, and sexual identity. A new world had opened up.

It wasn't long after that I began to reflect on my life before this "discovery." In fact, there had long been a disjuncture between my researcher identity and artist identity (in my case, as a writer of stories and poetry). My "work" had become compartmentalized. This process of reflection led me back to my earlier methods teachings: holistic approaches to research are not only about the epistemology–theory–methods nexus, but also *the relationship the researcher has with his or her work.* I knew that I needed to align my research, writing, and teaching, like some of the other scholars whose work I had been reading. I wanted my work to be unified and resonate with who I am within and beyond the academy.

The Turn to the Arts

The arts have always been an important part of my life, from the more than dozen years of ballet classes I took growing up, to my early days in college as a theater major, and my lifelong love of visual art that was cultivated by my mother who, like her father, is a painter. My daughter too fancies herself an artist, which has taken me to Boston's Museum of Fine Arts many Saturdays for the last couple of years—where, while waiting for her art classes to end, I wrote most of this book.

Through my teaching I have also become aware of the profound possibilities of the arts to jar people into seeing things differently, to transcend differences, and to foster connections. For example, over the years I have noticed in my Sociology of Gender course that after weeks

of reviewing feminist research on patriarchal violence, students are ulti-
matcly most moved when I bring in a video of feminist singer/songwriter
Tori Amos performing "Me and a Gun." I think what the arts most offers
and what traditional academic writing most fails to accomplish is *resonance.*

ABR practices have emerged out of the natural affinity between
research practice and artistic practice, both of which can be viewed as
crafts. Drawing on the capabilities of the creative arts, ABR practices offer
qualitative researchers alternatives to traditional research methods and
methodologies. *ABR practices are a set of methodological tools used by qualitative researchers across the disciplines during all phases of social research, including data collection, analysis, interpretation, and representation.* These emerging tools adapt the tenets of the creative arts in order to address social
research questions in *holistic* and *engaged* ways in which *theory and practice
are intertwined.* Arts-based practices draw on literary writing, music, performance, dance, visual art, film, and other mediums. Representational
forms include but are not limited to short narratives, novels, experimental
writing forms, poems, collages, paintings, drawings, performance scripts,
theater performances, dances, documentaries, and songs. Although a set
of methodological tools, this genre of methods also comprises new theoretical and epistemological groundings that are expanding the qualitative paradigm. As suggested in this book, ABR also *disrupts* traditional
research paradigms.

Why This Book Is Needed

I wrote this book as an in-depth introduction to ABR. Currently, there
are several wonderful books about various components of ABR, as well as
a comprehensive handbook. However, there are no introductory books
that cover the six genres reviewed in this text: narrative inquiry, poetry,
music, performance, dance/movement, and visual art. Furthermore,
this is the only book that pairs introductory chapters with empirical
research articles. It is my position that arts-based approaches to research
offer researchers new pathways for creating knowledge within and across
disciplinary boundaries from a range of epistemological and theoretical perspectives. These practices are congruent with critical perspectives on knowledge construction and many related methods practices
are particularly adept at accessing subjugated perspectives, challenging
stereotypes and dominant ideology, raising critical consciousness, fostering empathetic understandings, and building coalitions. ABR provides
researchers across the disciplines new ways to diversify the audiences for

their research. The goal of this book is to provide undergraduate and graduate students and scholars with alternative approaches to qualitative research and new ways for thinking about their artist–researcher–teacher identities.

Organization of This Book

This book pairs in-depth introductory chapters with empirical research articles written by leading ABR scholars. The pairing of the introductory review chapters with published research articles provides a context for understanding each arts-based innovation as well as empirical and theoretical examples of its use. The introductory chapters provide overviews of each methodological genre through the use of definitions of key terms, discussions of research design issues, examples of research questions and projects, the advantages of each methodological genre, and discussions of aesthetics, assessment, and representation. The research articles are meant to offer examples of how these methods have been used by scholars across the disciplines. With this said, some of the results of using the research practices reviewed in this book cannot be properly captured in a written text. For example, dance and creative movement cannot simply be transcribed textually. Similar issues are true for performance- as well as music-based methods. In research projects, these artistic formats either exist in the moment only or are partially retained via videotaping. With technological advances, many ABR practitioners now publish on the Internet, where they are able to stream video, archive sound files, and publish color imagery with far less expense than with traditional publishing. Therefore, the research articles following the introductory chapters should not be taken as full representations of how these methods are used, just partial examples.

The organization of this book mirrors one way of conceptualizing the journey of arts-based practices, as well as the interconnections between these methods, by following a *word to image* arch. In this vein, the first methodological genre covered, in Chapter 2, is narrative inquiry, which constitutes an extension of what many qualitative researchers already do. Narrative inquiry draws more explicitly on the arts than traditional qualitative research, but still relies on "the word" as its main communication tool and "(re)storying" as its mode of writing. Chapter 2 reviews the use of poetry in social research. Poetry merges "the word" with "lyrical invocation" and therefore represents both an extension of and a departure from traditional representational forms. Music as a method is explored in Chapter 4, picking up on the lyrical nature of poetry. As reviewed in

Chapter 4, this particular art form comes into being via performance; therefore, extending the tenets of music as method, Chapter 5 reviews performance-based methods of inquiry. As noted in this chapter, this vast methodological genre has exploded in recent decades, encompassing many methodological practices. Arguably, the most abstract form of performance is dance (or movement), which is the topic of Chapter 6. The final methods reviewed center on the visual arts, completing the arch *from word to image*.

Alternative Ways of Reading This Book

Although this book can be read in order, it need not be. Each introductory chapter can be read on its own; so too can the research articles. Therefore, readers who are interested in particular methodological genres can read just those pertinent chapters. Additionally, following the path from word to image was merely one way the book could be organized. Alternatively, some readers may view the "performance paradigm" as the major impetus for the call to the arts. In this vein, the separation of performance studies and dance/creative movement may be unnecessary. These readers may begin with those chapters. Finally, this book can be read in conjunction with a literature review on any of the topics covered. So, for example, a researcher or student interested in visual arts-based approaches to research may read the introductory chapter as well as Chapter 7 on visual arts alongside scholarly articles published in academic journals.

Audience for This Book

This book is accessibly written for diverse audiences including undergraduates, graduates, and scholars interested in methodology or ABR. Methodologists interested in innovative approaches to qualitative research or ABR will find this book useful. Although written for broad audiences, and appropriate for advanced undergraduate students, the book is also of value for those scholars who already employ ABR. Given the breadth of coverage, incorporation of research examples, and scholarly resources (discussed shortly), even methodologists who use ABR will likely benefit from the organization of this volume. In terms of teaching, this book can be used in courses in Sociology, Education, Social Work, Clinical Psychology, Communications, Health Studies, Theater Arts, and Women's Studies. It can be used as a primary text in Sociology of Art courses and as a supplemental text in courses including research methods, qualitative research, feminist research theory and methods, theater arts, performance studies, visual sociology, cultural studies, sociology of culture, and cultural anthropology.

Pedagogical Features and Resources

In addition to pairing in-depth introductory chapters with empirical research examples from noted scholars, numerous research examples are woven throughout each introductory chapter. Introductory chapters also note key terms and definitions, major methods within each methodological genre, and examples of research questions. The six chapters addressing the various arts-based methodological genres reviewed in this book also contain several special features. Each chapter ends with a checklist of considerations researchers should bear in mind as they contemplate using the particular methods reviewed. These checklists also provide guiding questions researchers can consider as they outline their own research design strategies. Researchers using this book will also find the annotated lists of suggested readings, journals, and websites located at the end of each chapter helpful. The annotated list of suggested readings allows researchers to further explore particular methodological practices, while the annotated lists of journals and websites provide avenues for expanding literature reviews as well as possible publishing venues for scholars working with arts-based practices. Finally, I have included a pedagogical feature professors can use as they teach with this text: discussion questions and activities that can be worked on collaboratively in class or assigned as homework. Researchers new to ABR may also find the activities useful as they get their hands wet with these new approaches to research.

Acknowledgments

In working toward completion of this book, I appreciate the help of a number of people who supported this endeavor. First and foremost, I thank my friend and editor extraordinaire, C. Deborah Laughton. I am grateful to Jennifer DePrima for her careful copy-edit of the manuscript, Laura Specht Patchkofsky for shepherding the book through production, and the staff at The Guilford Press for their enthusiastic support. I thank Natalie Graham in particular for assisting with this publication. I extend a spirited thank-you to my amazing research assistants, Ashley

Garland, Jillian Klotz, Kathryn Maloney, and Nathan Regan. Kathryn conducted extensive research on arts-based methods, which is incorporated throughout the book. Ashley, Jillian, and Nathan assisted with the manuscript preparation and provided assistance with the literature review and references. Thank you, Maryjean Viano Crowe, for allowing me to use your inspirational visual art—your work speaks to me deeply. I am also grateful for the support I have received from the staff and administration of Stonehill College. In particular, I thank Katie Conboy, Kathy Conroy, and Bonnie Troupe. A spirited thank-you to the reviewers whose comments have greatly clarified my thinking about ABR practices: Carolyn Ellis, PhD, Professor of Communications, University of South Florida, and Lynn Butler-Kisber, PhD, Associate Professor in the Department of Integrated Studies in Education at McGill University. In this vein, I extend a special thank-you again to Carolyn Ellis—the beauty of your writing is matched by the fullness of your spirit. Thank you, Carol Bailey—you are so generous; you must be an amazing teacher, and I am very grateful for your insights. I also extend my appreciation to Sharlene Hesse-Biber of Boston College—thank you for your mentorship in research methodology. Finally, I dedicate this book to my mother, Sylvia, and my daughter, Madeline. Mom, thank you for instilling in me a lifelong love of the arts and for telling me to write. And thank you for all of those magical lunches at the museum, a tradition Madeline and I now share. Madeline, you are my heart.

I am grateful to the publishers and authors for permission to reprint the following journal articles:

"What Kind of Mother . . . ?: An Ethnographic Short Story" by Karen Scott-Hoy (2002). Originally published in *Qualitative Inquiry*, *8*(3). Reprinted with permission from Sage Publications, Inc., Thousand Oaks, CA.

"Research as Poetry: A Couple Experiences HIV" by Cynthia Cannon Poindexter (2002). Originally published in *Qualitative Inquiry*, *8*(6). Reprinted with permission from Sage Publications, Inc., Thousand Oaks, CA.

"The Role of Music in an Art-Based Qualitative Inquiry" by Norma Daykin (2004). Reprinted with permission from the author and *International Journal of Qualitative Methods*, *3*(2). Available online at *www.ualberta.ca/~iiqm/backissues/3_2/pdf/daykin.pdf*.

"Exploring Risky Youth Experiences: Popular Theatre as a Participatory Performative Research Method" by Diane Conrad (2004). Reprinted with permission from the author and *International Jour-*

nal of Qualitative Methods, 3(1). Available online at *www.ualberta. ca/~iiqm/backissues/3_1/pdf/conrad.pdf.*

"Writing Rhythm: Movement as Method" by Mary Beth Cancienne and Celeste N. Snowber (2003). Originally published in *Qualitative Inquiry,* 9(2). Reprinted with permission from Sage Publications, Inc., Thousand Oaks, CA.

"Visual Portraits: Integrating Artistic Process into Qualitative Research" by Carolyn Jongeward (1997). Originally published in *Canadian Review of Art Education,* 24(2). Reprinted with permission from the author and the *Canadian Review of Art Education,* Toronto, Ontario, Canada.

The following works of art appear in this book with permission from the artist, Maryjean Viano Crowe: "Doll Cake 1," "Doll Cake 2," "Pie in the Sky," "The Bake Off," "Visions Danced in Her Head," "Coffee Crumbs," and "Cake Walk."

Contents

CHAPTER 1

Social Research
and the Creative Arts
An Introduction

> The most beautiful thing we can experience is the mysterious. It is
> the source of all true art and science.
> —ALBERT EINSTEIN

Many researchers in the social and behavioral sciences enter the academy full of what my mother calls "chutzpah": a palpable energy, desire to
make a difference, and fearlessness about shaking things up. Chutzpah
flows from passion. However, operating within a context of institutional
pressures of tenure and promotion clocks, coupled with publish-or-perish
dictates and funding agencies that reward "hard-science" practitioners,
many academics soon become disenchanted. They tell themselves that
they'll simply do the work they want to do later, which works because
"later" never arrives. Although traditional methods grounded in the
scientific method suit some, and traditional qualitative research methods create a working space for others, still there are the *other* others for
whom these research conventions make what was once a passion start to
feel more like a job.

Arts-based researchers are not "discovering" new research tools, they
are *carving* them. And with the tools they sculpt, so too a space opens
within the research community where passion and rigor boldly intersect
out in the open. Some researchers have come to these methods as a way
of better addressing research questions while some quite openly long to

1

merge their scholar-self with their artist-self. In all cases, whether in the particular arts-based project or in the researcher who routinely engages with these practices, a *holistic, integrated perspective* is followed.

In his eloquent book *A Methodology of the Heart: Evoking Academic and Daily Life,* Ronald Pelias (2004) writes: "I speak the heart's discourse because the heart is never far from what matters. Without the heart pumping its words, we are nothing but an outdated dictionary, untouched" (p. 7). In my own research on collective memory and national identity (see Leavy, 2007) I often felt that the "scraps" of data left strewn across my office floor were a part of the heart—the heart of my work and even more so the heart of my relationship with my work. As researchers, we are often trained to hide our relationship to our work; this is problematic for some, impossible for others. Arts-based research practices allow researchers to share this relationship with the audiences who consume their works. In Chapter 2 my short writing entitled "Fish Soup" illustrates, in a small way, what a research "scrap" can generate.

Pelias notes that arts-based texts are "methodological calls, writings that mark a different space. They collect in the body: an ache, a fist, a soup" (2004, p. 11). The turn to the creative arts in social research results from a confluence of many historically specific phenomena. Concurrently, these practices open up a new space that, as the negative space that defines a positive object in visual art, creates new ways of thinking about traditional research practices. What is clear when compiling recent arts-based research, and researchers' reflections on it, is that the pioneers in this area seek to sculpt engaged, holistic, passionate research practices that bridge and not divide both the artist-self and researcher-self with the researcher and audience and researcher and teacher. Researchers working with these new tools are merging their interests while creating knowledge based on resonance and understanding.

Art and science bear intrinsic similarities in their attempts to illuminate aspects of the human condition. Grounded in exploration, revelation, and representation, art and science work toward advancing human understanding. Although an artificial divide has historically separated our thinking about art and scientific inquiry, a serious investigation regarding the profound relationship between the arts and sciences is under way. This book reviews and synthesizes the merging of cross-disciplinary social research with the creative arts. In recent decades a new methodological genre has emerged at the intersections of multiple disciplines and disciplinary practices: arts-based research practices.

Arts-based research practices are a set of methodological tools used by qualitative researchers across the disciplines during all phases of social research, including data collection, analysis, interpretation, and representation. These emerging tools adapt the tenets of the creative arts in order to address social research questions in holistic and engaged ways in which theory and practice are intertwined. Arts-based methods draw on literary writing, music, performance, dance, visual art, film, and other mediums. Representational forms include but are not limited to short narratives, novels, experimental writing forms, poems, collages, paintings, drawings, performance scripts, theater performances, dances, documentaries, and songs. This genre of methods also comprises new theoretical and epistemological groundings that are expanding the qualitative paradigm.

A/r/tographical work is a specific category of arts-based research practices within education research. A/r/t is a metaphor for artist-researcher–teacher. In a/r/tography these three roles are integrated creating a *third space* (Pinar, 2004, p. 9). These practitioners occupy "in-between" space (Pinar, 2004, p. 9). A/r/tography merges "knowing, doing, and making" (Pinar, 2004, p. 9).

A group of Faculty of Education at the University of British Columbia began responding to a trend in research conducted largely by their graduate students, ultimately compiling a collection of more than 30 dissertations that used arts-based research. The faculty then analyzed the collection, identifying three major pillars of practice: literary, visual, and performative (Sinner, Leggo, Irwin, Gouzouasis, & Grauer, 2006). Additionally, this group uses the term "practices" instead of the more conventional term "methods" (Sinner et al., 2006, p. 1229), which in part signifies the break with methods conventions and also rejects the idea of tools that are neutrally implemented. Referring to a/r/tographical research as a localized and evolving methodology, Sinner and colleagues (2006) posit this is a "hybrid, practice-based form of methodology" (p. 1224) that is necessarily about both the self and the social. They write:

> A/r/tographical work is rendered through the methodological concepts of contiguity, living inquiry, openings, metaphor/metonymy, reverberations, and excess which are enacted and presented or performed when a relational aesthetic inquiry condition is envisioned as embodied understandings and exchanges between art and text, and between and among the broadly conceived identities of artist/researcher/teacher. (p. 1224)

For the remainder of this book I employ the umbrella category "arts-based research" as a way of including the fundamental tenets of a/r/tographical research.

This new breed of qualitative methods offers researchers alternatives to traditional research methods that may fail to "get at" the particular issues they are interested in, or may fail to represent them effectively. For example, the a/r/tographical research dissertation collection at the University of British Columbia includes research on the following topics: love, death, power, memory, fear, loss, desire, hope, and suffering (Sinner et al., 2006, p. 1238). These highly conceptual topics, which represent some of the most fundamental aspects of human experience, are often impossible to access through traditional research practices.

Alhough art has long been a subject for investigation in anthropology and art education, as well as other disciplines, only recently have the methodological *tools* employed in the arts been vigorously explored by social scientists, health care researchers, education researchers and practitioners, and others in order to reveal tremendous meaning-making and pedagogical capabilities. Although the arts are most typically associated in social research with the *representation stage* of research, as evidenced throughout this book, the arts are being used during *all phases* of the research endeavor from data collection to analysis and representation, as well as continuing to serve as a subject of inquiry and a pedagogical tool.

In this chapter I review the historical context in which arts-based methods have emerged; how they sit with respect to ontological, epistemological, theoretical, and methodological questions; the impact of these new strategies on the qualitative paradigm; and the primary reasons why a researcher might opt for an arts-based practice. In terms of the latter, I address the questions: What do these methods help us to unearth, illuminate, or present that would otherwise remain untapped or opaque? Why use an arts-based method as opposed to a traditional qualitative method? Finally, I review the organization of this book.

Pushing on the Borders of an Alternative Paradigm: Historical Context for Arts-Based Research

In order to understand how researchers have developed arts-based methodological practices they must be situated in a discussion of the emergence of the qualitative paradigm as an alternative to the quantitative paradigm. It is important to note that there are many competing ways to conceptualize qualitative research. I use the term "paradigm" to encompass the diverse expanse of qualitative research, which is practiced from many different epistemological and theoretical perspectives. I consider arts-based research to constitute a new methodological genre within the ever-evolving qualitative paradigm. I should also mention that although many qualitative researchers resent the endless comparisons of qualitative practices to quantitative practices (and rightfully so), given the historical dominance of quantitative research and the extent to which positivist approaches to evaluation remain "the gold standard," this kind of comparison seems warranted. Moreover, although this book is about a new genre of qualitative research practices, quantitative and qualitative methods are simply different approaches to answering social research questions.

Positivist Science

Positivist science, also referred to as empiricism, emerged in the late 1800s out of European rationalist movements. This model, first established in the natural sciences, is based on the "scientific method," and served as the foundation upon which social science perspectives on knowledge-building developed, largely as a result of the pioneering classical sociologist Emile Durkheim's effort to legitimize sociology by modeling the discipline after physics. With the publication of Durkheim's (1938/1965) book *The Rules of the Sociological Method*, which posited that the social world consisted of universal "social facts" that could be studied through objective, empirical means, positivist science crossed disciplinary boundaries and became the model for all scientific research.

The scientific method, which guides "hard science," developed out of a positivist ontological and epistemological viewpoint. Positivist science holds several basic beliefs about the nature of knowledge, which together form *positivist epistemology*, the cornerstone of the quantitative paradigm (Hesse-Biber & Leavy, 2005). Positivism holds that a knowable reality exists independently of the research process and this reality consists of knowable "truth," which can be discovered, measured, and controlled via the objective means employed by neutral researchers. Positivist science employs *deductive* methods. Within this framework, both the researcher and methodological instruments are presumed to be "objective." Like the natural world, the social world is governed by rules that result in patterns, and thus causal relationships between variables can be identified, hypotheses tested and proven, and causal relationships explained. Moreover, social reality is predictable and potentially controllable. The positivist view of social reality (the ontological question), researchers' objective and authoritative study of it (the epistemological question), and the tools designed to quantitatively measure and test the social world (methods) together comprise the quantitative paradigm (Hesse-Biber & Leavy, 2005). As noted by Thomas Kuhn (1962), a paradigm is a worldview through which knowledge is filtered.

For more than half a century diverse scholars have been challenging the basic tenets of positivism, resulting in an alternative worldview: the qualitative paradigm. *Qualitative research* is the term used to designate a diverse range of methods and methodological practices informed by various epistemological and theoretical groundings.

It is necessary to review the primary social and academic catalysts responsible for the major challenges to positivist science and eventual culmination into the qualitative paradigm (although such a brief history is certainly partial). Understanding this historical shift is directly related to contemplating the newer category of arts-based research practices because the main concern levied against these methods centers on issues of validity and trustworthiness. These evaluation concepts, however, were initially conceived in relation to the positivist perspective on knowledge-building and corresponding methods practices. As researchers working within the qualitative paradigm realized decades ago, the conventional strategies available for checking validity, reliability, and the like, as well as the appropriateness of these concepts, required new methods for achieving trustworthiness and new concepts that properly identified the benchmarks against which scientific "success" could be measured. Many argue that qualitative research is still at times mistakenly judged in quantitative terms and the legitimacy of qualitative evaluation techniques continue to be critiqued more than their quantitative counterparts. The resistance, by some, to the newer breed of arts-based practices is therefore linked to these larger struggles about scientific standards and knowledge-building. With this said, I turn to a brief review of the move toward qualitative research.

The Qualitative Paradigm

Qualitative research is generally characterized by *inductive* approaches to knowledge-building. Ethnography has long been the methodological cornerstone of anthropology, a discipline committed to studying people from various cultures in their natural settings. The shift toward ethnography across the disciplines largely emerged at the University of Chicago. In the 1920s researchers at the "Chicago School of Sociology" began using ethnography and related methods to study various hidden dimensions of urbanization in the area (among other topics). This in part prompted the use of qualitative methods in sociology departments around the United States, as well as the development of new theoretical perspectives that would further propel qualitative innovation. Ethnography produced what Clifford Geertz (1973) later termed "thick descriptions" of social life from the perspective of research participants (as well as the researcher's own interpretation of what he or she learns in the field). Moreover, this method required the researcher to develop rapport with his or her research participants, collaborate with them, and embark on weighty and unpredictable emotional as well as intellectual processes. Ethnography clearly challenges positivist assumptions about social reality and our study of it, making the use of this method outside of anthropology pivotal. Similarly, sociologists and health care researchers in the 1940s adapted the focus-group interview method that developed as a tool for then-burgeoning market researchers to suit a range of other topics.

Qualitative research was further propelled in 1959 with the publication of Erving Goffman's groundbreaking book *The Presentation of Self in Everyday Life*. In this work Goffman co-opted Shakespeare's famous line "all the world is a stage" and developed the term *dramaturgy* to denote the ways in which social life can be conceptualized as a series of ongoing performances complete with "front stage" and "backstage" behaviors, daily rituals of "impression management," including "face-saving behavior," and other ways in which people operate as *actors* on life's stage. Not only did Goffman's work move qualitative research forward at the time, but as reviewed in Chapter 5 on performance studies, his work has been foundational for more recent arts-based innovations.

More than any single work, the social justice movements of the 1960s and 1970s—the civil rights movement, the women's movement (second-wave feminism), the gay rights movement—culminated in major changes in the academic landscape, including the asking of new research questions as well as the reframing of many previously asked research questions and corresponding approaches to research, both theoretical and methodological. Populations such as women and people of color, formerly rendered invisible in social research or included in ways that reified stereotypes and justified relations of oppression, were sought out for meaningful inclusion. The common outgrowth from these diverse and progressive movements included a thorough reexamination of *power within the knowledge-building process* in order to avoid creating knowledge that continued to be complicit in the oppression of minority groups. This collective goal can metaphorically be conceptualized as a new tree trunk out of which many branches have grown.

For example, feminists developed standpoint epistemology as a means of acknowledging that a hierarchical social order produces different "standpoints" (experiences and corresponding perspectives), and standpoint epistemology spawned corresponding feminist methodologies (see Harding, 1993; Hartsock, 1983; Hill-Collins, 1990; Smith, 1987). Through their attention to power dynamics in the research process, many feminists also began a critical discourse about related issues and practices such as voice, authority, disclosure, representation, and reflexivity. Moreover, many argued that feminism should seek to produce "partial and situated truths" (see Haraway, 1988) and that feminists should be attentive to the "context of discovery" and not only the "context of justification," the focus in positivist research (see Harding, 1993). In these and other ways, feminists called for a dismantling of the dualisms on which positivism hinges: subject–object, rational–emotional, and concrete–abstract (Sprague & Zimmerman, 1993). Moreover, feminists challenged the positivist conception of "objectivity" that permeates positivist research practices. In this regard, feminists have argued that the positivist view of objectivity has produced a legacy of "scientific oppression"—relegating women, people of color, sexual minorities, and the disabled to the category of "other" (Halpin, 1989). All of these epistemological and theoretical advances prompted the increased interdisciplinary use of qualitative methods such as ethnography and oral history interview.

In addition to feminism and other social justice movements, globalization and a changing media and economic landscape influenced alternative theoretical schools of thought, including postmodernism, poststructuralism, postcolonialism, critical race theory, queer studies, and psychoanalysis (which also informs embodiment theory). All of these theoretical perspectives attend to issues of power and have caused a significant renegotiation and elaboration of the qualitative paradigm. For example, postmodern theory (an umbrella term for a diverse body of theories) rejects totalizing or "grand" theories, calls for a critical restructuring of "the subject," pays attention to the productive aspects of the symbolic realm, accounts for the sociopolitical nature of experience, and rejects essentialist identity categories that erase differences.

These theoretical and epistemological claims bear directly on methodological practices and the expansion of the qualitative paradigm. With the goal of troubling dominant knowledges or "jamming the theoretical machinery" (Irigaray, 1985, p. 78), researchers informed by postmodern and poststructural theories have adapted qualitative methods in order to expose and subvert oppressive power relations. For example, poststructuralists influenced by Jacques Derrida (1966) apply "deconstruction" and "discourse analysis" approaches to qualitative content analysis. Postmodern theorists have also brought issues of representation to the forefront of methodological debate. Arguing that form and content are inextricably bound and enmeshed within shifting relations of power (see Foucault, 1976), postmodernists have been integral to the advancement of arts-based methods of representation.

The qualitative paradigm has expanded greatly as a result of all of these advances in theory. It is within this politically, theoretically, and methodologically diverse paradigm that, in recent decades, arts-based practices have emerged as an alternative methodological genre.

Arts-Based Practices:
Disrupting and Extending the Qualitative Paradigm

A major shift in academic research began in the 1970s, and by the 1990s arts-based practices constituted a new methodological genre (Sinner et al., 2006, p. 1226). This shift is in part the result of work done in arts-based therapies. Health care researchers, special education researchers, psychologists, and others have increasingly turned to the arts for their therapeutic, restorative, and empowering qualities. Although there are differences between therapeutic practices and research practices, the work of these practitioners is cited throughout this text, as there is no doubt that knowledge derived from the practices of arts-based therapies has informed our understanding of arts-based research practices.

Although arts-based practices are an extension of the qualitative paradigm, these methods practices have posed serious challenges to qualitative methods conventions, thus unsettling many assumptions about what constitutes research and knowledge. Sava and Nuutinen (2003) refer to these methods as presenting a "troubling model of qualitative inquiry into self, art, and method" (p. 517). These disruptions to traditional research practices, much like early responses to the qualitative challenge to positivism, have caused concerns and inspired debates. As our methods history shows, such debates are critical to scientific progress, as they create a space for a professional public renegotiation of disciplinary practices and standards. Influenced by Elliot W. Eisner (1997), I therefore suggest that the emergence of arts-based social research advances critical conversations about the nature of social scientific practice and expands the borders of our methods repository. Eisner (1997) articulates the fear experienced by some as the methods borders are pushed making way for artistic representation.

> We have ... concretized our view of what it means to know. We prefer our knowledge solid and like our data hard. It makes for a firm foundation, a secure place on which to stand. Knowledge as a process, a temporary state, is scary to many. (p. 7)

It is important to remember that this trepidation parallels the fear quantitatively trained researchers expressed when qualitative research was emerging and struggling for legitimacy. In this regard, Jones (2006) notes that "novelty is always uncomfortable" (p. 12).

The move toward arts-based practices flows from several related issues. In this chapter I first address the nature of art and artists and the intrinsic parallels between artistic practice and the practice of qualitative research. Second, I address the strengths of arts-based practices. What kinds of research questions can be answered via these methods? What can these methods reveal and represent that cannot be captured with traditional qualitative methods? How can these methods be applied to access subjugated voices? Finally, I consider issues of assessment. How can knowledge constructed with these methods be evaluated? What are the primary dimensions of evaluation, and what methods strategies are currently available? How do these practices move conversations about knowledge construction forward?

Artistic and Social Scientific Practice

Both artistic practice and the practice of qualitative research can be viewed as *crafts*. Qualitative researchers do not simply gather and write; they *compose, orchestrate,* and *weave*. As Valerie J. Janesick (2001) notes, the researcher is the instrument in qualitative research as in artistic practice. Moreover, both practices are holistic and dynamic, involving reflection, description, problem formulation and solving, and the ability to identify and explain intuition and creativity in the research process. Therefore Janesick refers to qualitative researchers as "artist-scientists." She also suggests that if we begin to better understand and disclose how we use creativity and intuition in our research, then we can better understand the function of qualitative research. In this vein, a systematic exploration of arts-based practices can lead to a refining of the work we as qualitative researchers *already do.*

Hunter, Lusardi, Zucker, Jacelon, and Chandler (2002) similarly argue, from their perspective as health care researchers, that the creative arts can help qualitative researchers pay closer attention to how the complex process of meaning-making and idea percolation shapes research. Hunter and colleagues posit that although meaning-making is of course central to the research process, the "incubation phase" in qualitative research—the phase in which structured "intellectual chaos" occurs so that patterns may emerge and novel conclusions can be drawn—is given lip service but isn't actually legitimized as a distinct phase of the research process and is accordingly rushed through and later glossed over (p. 389). Hunter and colleagues suggest that the legitimized research process consists of the following four stages: (1) problem identification, (2) literature review, (3) methods, and (4) results (p. 389). Nevertheless, in qualitative research praxis the meaning-making process occurs as an *iterative process* (not a linear one) and meaning emerges through labeling, identifying, and classifying emerging concepts; interrelating concepts and testing hypotheses; finding patterns; and generating theory (p. 389). Furthermore, there is an interface between interpretation and analysis—the process is *holistic* (Hesse-Biber & Leavy, 2004, 2006b; Hunter et al., 2002). Hunter and colleagues argue that visual and other arts-based methods make this process explicit—allowing qualitative researchers to better accomplish what they already do—arts-based practices draw out the meaning-making process and push it to the forefront.

The move by qualitative researchers to the arts is not surprising to researchers in drama education, who note, for example, profound similarities between theater arts and qualitative inquiry. Joe Norris (2000) notes that in both fields there is an ongoing process of reexamining content in order to create new meanings, and that drama students constantly test hypotheses via "the magic of what if" (p. 41). Johnny Saldaña (1999) asserts that theater practitioners and qualitative researchers share many critical characteristics, including keen observational skills, analytic skills, storytelling proficiency, and the ability to think conceptually, symbolically, and metaphorically. Moreover, as indicated, both practices require creativity, flexibility, and intuition, and result in the communication of information from which an audience generates meaning. Saarnivaara (2003) posits that it is assumed there is a "chasm" separating social inquiry and artistic practice, in which the former is viewed as a conceptual arena and the latter as experiential. However, Saarnivaara suggests that this is an artificial dualism and that art and inquiry can be merged because they already entail a similar process. Saarnivaara writes about artists as follows:

> I am using the word *artist,* following Juha Varto (2001), in a loose sense—metaphorically—to describe a person who confronts her experiential world by means of a craft and without exerting any conscious conceptual influence and who draws on it to create something new. (p. 582)

Although some may argue that it is unrealistic to assume researchers are not applying conceptual frames, Saarnivaara makes an excellent point regarding the common theme of investigating experiential reality via a craft—a *process*, as opposed to the clearly graded stages that comprise quantitative inquiry.

In addition, the writing of qualitative research, as with the work of artists, is ultimately about (re)presenting a set of meanings to an audience. In this regard, Diaz (2002) writes, "The act of writing assumes an attitude of persuasiveness. Literary persuasion, or rhetoric, like much of visual persuasion, is artistic. As writers and painters we try to persuade our readers and viewers to see the world through our eyes" (p. 153). The arts simply provide qualitative researchers a broader palette of investigative and communication tools with which to garner and relay a range of social meanings. Moreover, the artists' palette provides tools that can serve and expand the promise of qualitative research.

Finally, technological advances have assisted with the development of arts-based innovations. Quite simply, new technologies have allowed for the construction, preservation, and dissemination of many new kinds of "texts." Examples of relevant technologies include the Internet, PhotoShop, digital cameras, digital imaging technology, and sound files. Actually, this is a point of difficulty with compiling this volume as a textual representation. Many of the methods used in this book either create data or representations that cannot be held on to, such as dance, or they create data that cannot be textually transcribed without losing the very essence the method seeks to reveal, such as music or performance. These new technologies therefore allow researchers to use the arts in ways not previously possible. The Internet is particularly important for the dissemination of arts-based research.

Given the similarities between artistic practice and qualitative research, what are the methodological possibilities associated with arts-based practices?

The Strengths of Arts-Based Research Practices

Interdisciplinary arts-based practices have developed to service all phases of the research endeavor: data collection, analysis, interpretation, and representation. Many researchers referred to in this volume suggest that an artistic method, such as visual art or performance, can serve as an entire methodology in a given study. Moreover, arts-based practices allow research questions to be posed in new ways, entirely new questions to be asked, and new nonacademic audiences to be reached.

Arts-based practices are particularly useful for research projects that aim to *describe, explore,* or *discover.* Furthermore, these methods are generally attentive to *processes.* The capability of the arts to capture process mirrors the unfolding nature of social life, and thus there is a congruence between subject matter and method. Liora Bresler discusses this in detail and is referred to in Chapter 4, which explores music-based practices.

The arts, at their best, are known for being emotionally and politically evocative, captivating, aesthetically powerful, and moving. Art can grab people's attention in powerful ways. The arresting power of "good" art, whether musical, performance-based, or visual, is intimately linked with the *immediacy* of art (the concept of "good art" itself needs modification with respect to arts-based practice and this is discussed shortly). These are some of the qualities that qualitative researchers are harnessing in their arts-based research projects.

As a representational form, the arts can be highly effective for communicating the emotional aspects of social life. For example, theatrical representations of the experience of homelessness, the experience of living with a debilitating illness, or surviving sexual assault can get at elements of the lived experience that a textual form cannot reach. Furthermore, the dramatic presentation connects with audiences on a deeper, more emotional level and can thus evoke compassion, empathy, and sympathy, as well as understanding. In this way, arts-based practices can be employed as a means of creating *critical awareness* or *raising consciousness*. This is important in social justice–oriented research that seeks to reveal power relations (often invisible to those in privileged groups), raise critical race or gender consciousness, build coalitions across groups, and challenge dominant ideologies.

Arts-based practices are often useful in studies involving *identity work*. Research in this area often involves communicating information about the experiences associated with differences, diversity, and prejudice. Moreover, identity research seeks to confront stereotypes that keep some groups disenfranchised while other groups are limited by their own biased "common-sense" ideas. For example, Sandra L. Faulkner (2006) conducted in-depth interviews with people who are Jewish and lesbian, gay, or bisexual. This interview research, discussed in detail in Chapter 3 on poetry, is particularly interesting because Faulkner elected to conduct identity work with people who occupy two concealable identities—identities that may also conflict with each other. Part of her research centers on how her respondents chose to reveal or conceal their Jewish identity and sexual identity in different contexts. In order to most effectively communicate the powerful themes that emerged from her interviews, Faulkner used a poetic form of data representation. As with most identity-based research, part of the goal is to communicate the data in such a way as to challenge stereotypes, build empathy, promote awareness, and stimulate dialogue.

Faulkner's research also brings us to the next dimension of raising awareness: *giving voice to subjugated perspectives*. Many qualitative researchers, particularly those influenced by the theoretical perspectives that emerged from the social justice movements of the 1960s and 1970s, are interested in accessing subjugated voices. In other words, many qualitative researchers across the disciplines seek to give voice to those who have been marginalized as a result of their race, ethnicity, gender, sexual orientation, nationality, religion, disability, or other factors (as well as the interconnections between these categories). For example, as noted in Chapter 6 on dance as a method, Carol Picard's (2000) research on the effectiveness of movement as a part of a multimethod research design centered in accessing personal narratives from women at midlife, whose stories have long been silenced in scientific research and made invisible in mainstream culture.

Arts-based practices can also *promote dialogue*, which is critical to cultivating understanding. The particular ways in which art forms facilitate conversation are important as well. The arts ideally evoke emotional responses, and so the dialogue sparked by arts-based practices is highly engaged. By connecting people on emotional and visceral levels, artistic forms of representation facilitate empathy, which is a necessary precondition for challenging harmful stereotypes (pertinent in identity research) and building coalitions/community across differences (pertinent in action research and other projects with activist components). For example, in Chapter 4 I note Stacy Holman Jones's (2002) research on torch singing as a method of bringing women together despite racial and economic differences. By accessing subjugated voices and promoting dialogue, these methods are very useful for unsettling dominant stereotypes and providing people with the tools necessary (such as compassion) to continue problematizing dominant ideologies. In this vein, these methods serve postmodern attempts at subversion.

In addition, the use of arts-based representational strategies brings academic scholarship to a wider audience. Free from discipline-specific jargon and other prohibitive (even elitist) barriers, arts-based representations can be shared with diverse audiences, expanding the effect of scholarly research that traditionally circulates within the academy and arguably does little to serve the public good. In this vein, with *public sociology* on the rise, arts-based practices may continue to see an increase as a result of their representational strengths. It is important to remember that the capability of arts-based texts to reach diverse audiences is, at this point, largely an ideal that has yet to be realized. Given the pressures to publish and present research, many scholars who use these methods present their research at scholarly conferences and publish in alternative academic journals, thus limiting the public nature of the results. Nevertheless, the possibility for wider dissemination is there.

The kind of dialogue promoted by arts-based practices is predicated upon *evoking meanings*, not denoting them. In other words, although qualitative research typically claims to be inductive by design, it often falls short with preconceived language, code categories, and guiding assumptions creeping into the process, often more than we may realize. Arts-based practices lend themselves to *inductive* research designs. In this way, these methods again can be viewed as mirroring the ideal goals of conventional qualitative research and offering new tools to facilitate these goals.

The inductive nature of these methods is connected with the strength of arts-based practices to get at *multiple meanings*. Qualitative researchers working from many perspectives are interested in accessing multiple meanings, which links back to the critique of positivism as a perspective that has historically concealed multiple meanings by proposing universal truths that have oppressed and silenced many groups, often rendering them invisible within knowledge production. This is one of the reasons that some researchers conducting identity research, for example, have turned to arts-based practices. The attention to multiplicity and inductive focus afforded by arts-based practices has affected their current popularity. Carl Bagley and Mary Beth Cancienne (2002) speak to this issue as they reflect on their use of dance as a representational form in their education research project.

> In "dancing the data" we were able to facilitate a movement away from and disruption of the monovocal and monological nature of the voice in the print-based paper. Through a choreographed performance we were provided with an opportunity to encapture the multivocal and dialogical, as well as to cultivate multiple meanings, interpretations, and perspectives that might engage the audience in a recognition of textual diversity and complexity. (p. 16)

Arts-based practices help qualitative researchers access and represent the multiple viewpoints made imperceptible by traditional research methods. For the many researchers committed to accessing subjugated voices, engaging in reflexive practice, and opening up a public discourse, arts-based practices are a welcome alternative to traditional modes of knowledge-building.

Struggles over Standards:
Validity, Assessment, Trustworthiness,
and the Renegotiation of Scientific Criteria

The emergence of arts-based practices has necessitated a renegotiation of the qualitative paradigm with respect to fundamental assumptions about scientific standards of evaluation. In particular, these methods have been interrogated around issues of validity, trustworthiness, and authenticity. Critics as well as those who practice arts-based research have asked: How can we evaluate knowledge constructed with these methods?

Traditional conceptions of validity and reliability, which developed out of positivism, are inappropriate for evaluating artistic inquiry. Unlike positivist approaches to social inquiry, arts-based practices produce partial, situated, and contextual truths. These innovations require a modification of traditional evaluation standards and a move away from "rigor" and toward "vigor" (Sinner et al., 2006, p. 1252). The aim of these approaches is resonance, understanding, multiple meanings, dimensionality, and collaboration. Pelias suggests that all research offers first-person narratives (2004, p. 7). He writes:

> Some would object: To say all research is first-person narrative is not to say that all research is about the heart. The heart pushes the self forward to places it doesn't belong.
>   And I would respond: I don't want to go places where the heart is not welcome. Such places frighten me.
>   Are you frightened by the truth? would come the rejoinder.
>   No, I'm frightened by what poses as the truth. (p. 8)

Perspectives on how to attain authentic and trustworthy results are grounded in a researcher's ontological and epistemological assumptions. There is no "one-size-fits-all" model of evaluation with respect to knowledge derived from qualitative methods. The "success" of any given research project is linked to the research purpose(s) and how well the methodology has facilitated research objectives and communicated research findings. Although there is no standardized approach to attaining trustworthiness, as there is in positivist science, there are many methods for achieving trustworthiness that should be considered during research design and ultimately built into the project.

Although qualitative methods of assessment may be useful in some instances, in others the new artistic methods require new, flexible methods of assessment or adaptations of more conventional approaches. In this way, artistic forms of social inquiry move conversations about knowledge construction forward. Although researchers are still working through many of the theoretical, methodological, and ethical issues to emerge from these new practices, there are strategies that can be incorporated at the point of research design. Issues surrounding evaluation are considered throughout this book as they pertain to particular methods; however, here I present a review of major assessment issues and strategies. These methods are linked to various dimensions of arts-based research.

Aesthetics

The issue of *aesthetics* is central to the production of arts-based texts as well as our evaluation of them. Although in the best cases art provokes, inspires, captivates, and reveals, certainly not all art can meet these standards. Throw novices into the mix who create art *for their scholarly research* and even less of what is produced is likely to meet the aesthetic ideals developed in the fine arts. Simultaneously, scholarly texts have rarely been judged on the basis of aesthetics, although in arts-based research this springs forth as a central feature of representation. There are two primary avenues for addressing the question of aesthetics in arts-based research: the theoretical and the methodological.

On a theoretical level, the emergence of these new methods necessitates not only a reevaluation of "truth" and "knowledge" but also of "beauty" (Jones, 2006, p. 1). Furthermore, the research community needs to expand the concepts of "good art" and "good research" to accommodate these methodological practices (Sinner et al., 2006, p. 1229). Piirto (2002) asks: What level of expertise in the particular art form being used must one have? While arts-based research texts must be rendered with consideration for the aesthetic qualities, so too must audiences or evaluators be cognizant that these are not "pure" artistic representations but rather *research texts*. The important assessment questions are: How does the work make one feel? What does the work evoke or provoke? What does the work reveal? In this vein, Leggo (2008) writes:

> The question shifts from "*Is this good arts-based research?*" to "*What is this arts-based research good for?*" The evaluation of the knowledge generated in arts-based research includes a critical investigation of the craft and aesthetics of artistic practices; a creative examination of how art evokes responses and connections; a careful inquiry into the methods that art uses to unsettle ossified thinking and provoke imagination; a conscientious consideration of the resonances that sing out to the world from word, image, sound, and performance. (quoted in Sinner et al., 2006, p. 1252, original emphasis)

In other words, aesthetic evaluation is based on the *value of the work* in terms of research and pedagogical functions (Sinner et al., 2006, p. 1252).

On a methodological level, it is necessary to recognize that the arts have different criteria for evaluating works as compared with the social and behavioral sciences. Faulkner (2005) urges researchers to merge scientific and artistic criteria in order to suit their hybrid arts-based methods. Faulkner also argues a related point, as does Percer (2002), both advocating that researchers *pay attention to the artistic craft* they are adapting and *learn the rules and tradition* they are borrowing from (and not simply assume that they can "dabble" in poetry, for example, without any research into the discipline itself). In this regard, cross-disciplinary collaborations are vital with respect to strengthening the aesthetic dimensions of research.

Interdisciplinary Collaboration and Reflection

Working with innovative methodologies often requires researchers to cross disciplinary boundaries, leave their comfort zones, and seek the expertise of researchers/practitioners in other areas (Hesse-Biber & Leavy, 2006a, 2008). In order to produce engaging texts Jones (2006, p. 4) advocates "cross-pollination." The best of arts-based practices calls on scholars to work with professionals outside their disciplines in order to maximize the aesthetic qualities and authenticity of the work. Moreover, the more effective the artistic aspects are, the more likely the research is to affect audiences in their intended ways.

Arts-based research often evokes emotional responses (intentionally) from audiences. Ascertaining information about audience response may therefore serve as another validity check (as well as a data source). Cho and Trent (2005) recommend getting feedback during all phases of the research project, a plan for which can be built into the research design. A variation on this is incorporating a specific "external review phase" or "external dialogue" in which experts, colleagues, or interested subpopulations are invited to consume the data and offer their feedback. Kip Jones (2006) uses *reflection teams* in his narrative analysis research, so that analysis is a collaborative process. Given that arts-based practices are often used as representational vehicles in social justice–oriented studies, many researchers have a postperformance or postviewing *dialogue with the audience.* During this time researchers can gauge how well appropriate emotions were evoked and that no harm was done. Additionally, researchers can assess how well other research objectives were met. For example, did the findings promote connections and community, increase awareness or consciousness, instigate political or social action, or inspire social justice across differences? Moreover, did the audience experience the representation as "truthful"? Did the audience have an unintended or worrisome response? For example, did audience members seem enraged, depressed, or otherwise adversely affected? What safeguards are in place to protect audience members?

Creating a space for dialogue with the audience is also vital to the negotiation of meanings and incorporation of multiple perspectives. As noted, accessing multiple meanings and integrating diverse perspectives is often a goal of qualitative research, and therefore building a dialogue into the research design facilitates this objective while also adding a dimension of validity to the data.

Subject–Object

Arts-based research practices change the traditional subject–object relationship (Sinner et al., 2006). Researchers using these methods are necessarily engaged, working on projects of import to both self and others (Sinner et al., 2006, p. 1238). In recent decades qualitative researchers influenced by feminism and other critical perspectives have claimed that researchers need to actively use and account for their emotions (and other aspects of subjective experience) in the research process (see Harding, 1993; Jaggar, 1989). The call to merge the rational–emotional and subject–object dichotomies challenges positivism, which teaches researchers to disavow their feelings. Because emotions play an important role in artistic expression they can also serve as important signals in the practice of arts-based methods. Researchers can use emotions as a "validity checkpoints." For example, researchers can engage in an "internal dialogue," as termed by Tenni, Smyth, and Boucher (2003), in which they monitor their emotional, psychological, carnal, and intellectual responses throughout the process. Keeping a diary, a practice similar to memo-writing in traditional ethnography, is one method for systematically engaging in this kind of internal dialogue (Tenni et al., 2003).

Theory

Researchers using arts-based practices of inquiry are also adapting traditional qualitative research design features in order to authenticate their research findings. *Using theory explicitly* during data analysis is one way to generate new interpretations and alternative meanings. For example, looking at a particular dataset through a multicultural lens allows the researcher to "see" things that might otherwise not stand out. Applying a macro perspective to data collected from individuals can help researchers situate individual biographies in the larger sociohistorical context, as is discussed in Chapter 2, with respect to autoethnography and narrative inquiry.

Literature Review

Literature reviews may also play an important role in arts-based research projects. As theory can be used to link micro and macro contexts, so too can existing scholarship be employed in this way. As some arts-based practices involve the explicit use of autobiographical data and/or fiction, literature reviews become a key source for adding multiple voices into the project, providing context and creating inferences. In addition, differing from conventional research practices, which typically start with a series of hypotheses and/or research questions, an arts-based project may stem from a literature review or other source (such as a work of art). Sinner and colleagues (2006) note that in some cases "sources [are] both the process and product of arts-based research" (p. 1242).

Analysis Cycles

In addition to using theory and existing scholarship during analysis, *engaging in cycles of analysis* throughout the research process, advocated by grounded-theory approaches to research, can also help researchers utilizing these methods to locate themselves within the process, cycle back to reexamine earlier interpretations, and better recognize the point of data saturation (Tenni et al., 2003). Traditional approaches such as *triangulation* can also be employed. Researchers can also highlight anomalies and juxtapose different data during representation in order to expose differences and contradictions. These strategies add to the trustworthiness of the data.

Ethics

As many researchers utilizing conventional qualitative research methods advocate, full *disclosure* with respect to methodological choices (both the context of discovery and context of justification) strengthens the resulting knowledge. Methodological disclosure is particularly important with arts-based practices as they struggle to find their place within the larger world of social inquiry. Arts-based practices such as short story writing may incorporate elements of fiction, making full methodological disclosure critical to an audience's understanding of a particular study as well as contributing to the legitimacy of knowledge constructed via artistic methods more generally.

The Organization of This Book: From Word to Image

Arts-based research practices open up a new range of research questions and topics, expand the diversity of audiences exposed to social research, and enrich the qualitative paradigm. This book explores six new areas of methodological innovation: narrative inquiry, poetry, music, performance, dance, and visual art. For each topic, I have written a chapter that reviews how the method developed, the methodological variations of the method, what kinds of research questions the practices can address, examples of studies conducted with the method, and other issues such as validity and representation. These chapters also include pedagogical features such as discussion questions and activities, as well as features designed for researchers, including checklists of considerations and annotated lists of journals, websites, and recommended readings. These features allow interested readers to pursue particular methodological innovations in greater depth and are also meant to assist researchers who wish to pursue scholarship with these methods.

This volume also includes previously published articles by scholars who have worked with the various methods covered. The pairing of the introductory review chapters with published research articles provides a context for understanding each arts-based innovation as well as empirical and theoretical examples of their use. With this said, some of the results of using the methods in this book cannot be properly captured in a written text. For example, dance and creative movement cannot be transcribed textually. In research projects these artistic formats either exist in the moment only, or are partially retained via videotaping. Similar issues are true for performance as well as music-based practices. Therefore the research articles following the introductory chapters should not be taken as full representations of how these methods are used. Researchers interested in working with these methods can, however, consider using the Internet as a site for storing and sharing sound files or streaming video. In this way, recordings of the results of performative methods can be made accessible in a way that traditional books or journals prevent. Many arts-based researchers also publish color imagery on the Internet at far less expense than traditional publishing.

Finally, the organization of the book mirrors one way of conceptualizing the journey of arts-based practices, as well as the interconnections between these practices. In this vein, Chapter 2 covers narrative inquiry, which constitutes an extension of what many qualitative researchers already do. Narrative inquiry draws more explicitly on the arts than traditional qualitative research, but still relies on "the word" as its main communication tool and "(re)storying" as its mode of writing. Chapter 3 reviews the use of poetry in social research. Poetry merges the word with "lyrical invocation" and therefore represents both an extension of and departure from traditional representational forms. Music as a method is explored in Chapter 4, picking up on the lyrical nature of poetry. Music comes into being via performance, and therefore extending the tenets of music as method, Chapter 5 reviews performance-based methods of inquiry. This vast methodological genre has exploded in recent decades, encompassing many methodological practices. Arguably, the most abstract form of performance is dance (or movement), which is the topic of Chapter 6. The final practices reviewed center on the visual arts (Chapter 7), completing the arc *from word to image.*

REFERENCES

Bagley, C., & Cancienne, M. B. (2002). Educational research and intertextual forms of (re)presentation. In C. Bagley & M. B. Cancienne (Eds.), *Dancing the data* (pp. 3–32). New York: Peter Lang.

Bresler, L. (2005). What musicianship can teach educational research. *Music Education Research, 7*(2), 169–183.

Cho, J., & Trent, A. (2005). *Process-based validity for performance-related qualitative work: Imaginative, artistic and co-reflexive criteria.* Pullman: Washington State University.

Derrida, J. (1966). The decentering event in social thought. In A. Bass (Trans.), *Writing the difference* (pp. 278–282). Chicago: University of Chicago Press.

Diaz, G. (2002). Artistic inquiry: On Lighthouse Hill. In C. Bagley & M. B. Cancienne (Eds.), *Dancing the data* (pp. 147–161). New York: Peter Lang.

Durkheim, E. (1965). *The rules of sociological method* (8th ed.) (S. A. Solovay & J. H. Mueller, Trans., & G. E. G. Catlin, Ed.). New York: Free Press. (Original work published 1938)

Eisner, E. W. (1997). The promise and perils of alternative forms of data representation, *Educational Researcher, 26*(6), 4–10.

Faulkner, S. L. (2006). Reconstruction: LGBTQ and Jewish. *Communication Annual, 29,* 95–120.

Foucault, M. (1976). Power as knowledge. In R. Hurley (Trans.), *The history of sexuality: Vol. 1. An introduction* (pp. 92–102). New York: Vintage Books.

Geertz, C. (1973). *The interpretation of cultures.* New York: Basic Books.

Goffman, E. (1959). *The presentation of self in everyday life.* Garden City, NY: Anchor.

Halpin, Z. (1989). Scientific objectivity and the concept of "the other." *Women's Studies International Forum, 12*(3), 285–294.

Haraway, D. (1988). Situated knowledges: The science question in feminism and the privilege of partial perspective. *Feminist Studies, 14,* 575–599.

Harding, S. (1993). Rethinking standpoint epistemology: What is "strong objectivity"? In L. Alcoff & E. Potter (Eds.), *Feminist epistemologies* (pp. 49–82). New York: Routledge.

Hartsock, N. (1983). The feminist standpoint: Developing the ground for a specifically feminist historical materialism. In S. Harding & M. Hintikka (Eds.), *Discovering reality* (pp. 283–305). Dordrecht, The Netherlands: Reidel.

Hesse-Biber, S. N., & Leavy, P. (2004). Distinguishing qualitative research. In S. N. Hesse-Biber & P. Leavy (Eds.), *Approaches to qualitative research: A reader on theory and practice* (pp. 1–15). New York: Oxford University Press.

Hesse-Biber, S. N., & Leavy, P. (Eds.). (2006a). *Emergent methods in social research.* Thousand Oaks, CA: Sage.

Hesse-Biber, S. N., & Leavy, P. (2006b) *The practice of qualitative research*. Thousand Oaks, CA: Sage.

Hesse-Biber, S. N., and Leavy, P. (2008). Pushing on the methodological boundaries: The growing need for emergent methods within and across the disciplines. In S. N. Hesse-Biber & P. Leavy (Eds.), *Handbook of emergent methods* (pp. 1–15). New York: Guilford Press.

Hill-Collins, P. (1990). Black feminist thought in the matrix of domination. In P. Hill-Collins, *Black feminist thought: Knowledge, consciousness, and the politics of empowerment* (pp. 221–238). Boston: Unwin Hyman.

Holman Jones, S. (2002). Emotional space: Performing the resistive possibilities of torch singing. *Qualitative Inquiry, 8*(6), 738–759.

Hunter, H., Lusardi, P., Zucker, D., Jacelon, C., & Chandler, G. (2002). Making meaning: The creative component in qualitative research. *Qualitative Health Research Journal, 12*(3), 388–398.

Irigaray, L. (1985). *This sex which is not one*. Ithaca, NY: Cornell University Press.

Jaggar, A. (1989). Love and knowledge: Emotion in feminist epistemology. *Inquiry, 32*, 151–172.

Janesick, V. J. (2001). Intuition and creativity: A pas de deux for qualitative researchers. *Qualitative Inquiry, 7*(5), 531–540.

Jones, K. (2006). A biographic researcher in pursuit of an aesthetic: The use of arts-based (re)presentations in "performative" dissemination of life stories. *Qualitative Sociology Review, 1*(2). *www.qualitativesociologyreview.org/ENG/index_eng.php*

Kuhn, T. (1962). *The structure of scientific revolutions*. Chicago: University of Chicago Press.

Leavy, P. (2007). *Iconic events: Media, politics and power in retelling history*. Lanham, MD: Lexington Books.

Leggo, C. (2008). Astonishing silence: Knowing in poetry. In J. G. Knowles & A. L. Cole (Eds.), *Handbook of the arts in qualitative social science research* (pp. 165–174). Thousand Oaks, CA: Sage.

Norris, J. (2000). Drama as research: Realizing the potential of drama in education as a research methodology. *Youth Theatre Journal, 14*, 40–51.

Pelias, R. J. (2004). *A methodology of the heart: Evoking academic and daily life*. Walnut Creek, CA: AltaMira Press.

Percer, L. H. (2002, June). Going beyond the demonstrable range in educational scholarship: Exploring the intersections of poetry and research. *Qualitative Report, 7*(2). Retrieved June 14, 2004, from *www.nova.edu/ssss/QR/QR7-2/hayespercer.html*

Picard, C. (2000). Patterns of expanding consciousness on midlife women. *Nursing Science Quarterly, 13*(2), 150–157.

Piirto, J. (2002). The question of quality and qualifications: Writing inferior poems as qualitative research. *International Journal of Qualitative Research in Education, 15*(4), 421–445.

Pinar, W. F. (2004). Foreword. In R. L. Irwin & A. de Cosson (Eds.), *A/r/tography: Rendering self through arts-based living inquiry* (pp. 9–25). Vancouver, BC: Pacific Educational Press.

Saarnivaara, M. (2003). Art as inquiry: The autopsy of an [art] experience. *Qualitative Inquiry, 9*(4), 580–602.

Saldaña, J. (1999). Playwriting with data: Ethnographic performance texts. *Youth Theatre Journal, 14,* 60–71.

Sava, I., & Nuutinen, K. (2003). At the meeting place of word and picture: Between art and inquiry. *Qualitative Inquiry, 9*(4), 515–534.

Sinner, A., Leggo, C., Irwin, R., Gouzouasis, P., & Grauer, K. (2006). Arts-based education research dissertations: Reviewing the practices of new scholars. *Canadian Journal of Education, 29*(4), 1223–1270.

Smith, D. (1987). *The everyday world as problematic: A feminist sociology.* Boston: Northeastern University Press.

Sprague, J., & Zimmerman, M. (1993). Overcoming dualisms: A feminist agenda for sociological method. In P. England (Ed.), *Theory on gender/feminism on theory* (pp. 255–279). New York: DeGruyter.

Tenni, C., Smyth, A., & Boucher, C. (2003). The researcher as autobiographer: Analyzing data written about oneself. *Qualitative Report, 8*(1): 1–12.

Varto, J. (2001). *Kauneuden taito* [*The craft of beauty*]. Tampere, Finland: Tampereen Yliopistopaino.

CHAPTER 2

⟡

Narrative Inquiry

Beauty is truth—truth, beauty—that is all Ye know on earth,
and all ye need to know.

—JOHN KEATS

Telling, retelling, writing, and rewriting stories are fundamental parts of social life and our study of it. As Clandinin and Connelly (1989) posit, narrative is not merely a method but a "basic phenomenon of life" (p. 2). The surge in narrative inquiry over the past few decades represents a shift from traditional qualitative methods to arts-based qualitative inquiry. Clandinin and Rosiek (2007) note that since the late 1960s, narrative inquiry has become increasingly common across the disciplines.

Writing is, and has always been, an integral part of social research, as it is necessarily entwined with the construction of knowledge. Moreover, language or "the word" has traditionally been the communicative device employed in the service of social scientific knowledge-building. Likewise, there is a rich tradition of storytelling methods in the qualitative paradigm that draw on cultural practices of oral knowledge transmission, such as oral history and life history. In this vein, the artistic turn to narrative in the social sciences can in many ways be viewed as the evolution of more conventional research practices and the naming and redefining of a wide set of practices.

Pinnegar and Daynes (2007) note four converging phenomena with respect to the turn to narrative inquiry. These four broad themes all pertain to the expansion of the qualitative paradigm and include (1) the relationship of the researched and researcher, (2) the move from numbers to words as data, (3) a shift from the general to the particular, and (4) the emergence of new epistemologies.

With regard to emergent epistemological views, or new ways of knowing, narrative inquiry has grown in relation to advances in post-modern theory, in particular within the context of serious investigations into the methodological implications of postmodern perspectives. Denzin (2001) has termed what he views as the "cinematic interview society" and has written extensively about reconstructing "the interview" as a way of creating "performance texts." In addition, postmodern scholarship has drawn attention to complex issues of embodiment and what Jones (2006) refers to as "embodied perception" (p. 8). Influenced by a postmodern sensibility, Jones argues that the surge in narrative inquiry is also linked to increased awareness of the role social science has in maintaining or resisting current relations of power. Jones advocates various forms of narrative inquiry as a way of creating "reflective and dialogic approaches of postmodern biographic social science" (p. 6) that reject the "codified language" historically used in academia and the limited venues in which that research circulates. When writing of the benefits of this perspective on narrative research he notes:

> Thus, our considerations, through embodied perception, encourage us to walk around the edges of stories, to see beyond factuality to the humanism hidden on the other side. By extending our gaze beyond the visual journals and books when seeking venues for dispersion of biographic studies, to new technologies and modes of presentation we open the doors to new understandings and resources. (p. 8)

In these ways the move toward narrative inquiry, complete with a set of aesthetic practices, is an extension of postmodern perspectives on the interview. Moreover, technological innovations, such as the Internet, enable the promise of postmodern theory to be more fully realized in empirical scholarship.

In this chapter I use the term "narrative inquiry" as an umbrella category for a variety of arts-based methodological practices involving storytelling and writing. Additionally, I consider applying nonfiction and fiction lenses to the research and writing process.

A *narrative* is, most simply put, a story. Moreover, a narrative is necessarily "*about something*" (Labov, 2006, p. 37, original emphasis). The sharing of narratives in daily life occurs when a person wants to tell others "about something" and that something is "an event—something that happened" (Labov, 2006, p. 38). Clandinin and Connelly (1989) are pioneers in the field of narrative inquiry in educational studies and suggest that the term "names a fundamental structure and quality of experience, both personal and social" (p. 2). In this regard, narrative can be viewed as a frame through which people make sense of their lives. Clandinin and Connelly note: "If ... we take the view that the storied quality of experience is both unconsciously and consciously restoried, retold and relived through processes of reflection, then the rudiments of method are born in the phenomenon of narrative" (p. 2). In its most basic form, narrative inquiry is "the description and restorying of the narrative structure" (Clandinin & Connelly, 1989, p. 2).

A *narrative perspective* changes the practice of traditional qualitative interviews. The *narrative method* is a collaborative method of telling stories, reflecting on stories, and (re)writing stories. This method can be employed during data collection and analysis and relies on traditional methods practices as well, commonly ethnographic observations and various forms of interviews or authoethnographic data (although documents and data in other forms can be incorporated into projects as well). The process of narrative inquiry demands that researchers pay attention to the fact that research participants are simultaneously telling and retelling their stories as they are living them (Clandinin & Connelly, 1989, p. 11). In this way, participants are engaged in the unfolding stories they share—stories that they restory or replot through their own reflective process and with the passing of time.

There are many ways to use narrative inquiry, not all of which can be discussed here. First I review several approaches that involve gathering data from participants via interviews and ethnographic observations as well as related analysis and writing procedures. Second I consider autoethnographic (or self-study) approaches to narrative studies. Finally I consider the explicit use of fiction as a research and writing tool.

- What is the narrative method?
- How can this approach be employed?
- What kinds of research questions is this method suited for?
- How are data analyzed?

Narrative Method

Building on the tenets of ethnography, oral history, and qualitative interview, the *narrative method* or *narrative inquiry* attempts to collaboratively access participants' life experiences and engage in a process of storying and restorying in order to reveal multidimensional meanings and present an authentic and compelling rendering of the data. In other words,

narratives are constructed out of the data through a reflexive, participatory, and aesthetic process. Research based on narrative inquiry produces arts-based writings. Narrative inquiry often relies on small sample
sizes but produces rich case studies.

As with the other methods reviewed in this volume, this kind of
research must be evaluated in relation to the goals and practices of the
method. Therefore positivist standards of validity and the like are inappropriate benchmarks of trustworthiness. Drawing on the groundbreaking work of Barone and Eisner (1997), Kim (2006) notes the following
qualities of arts-based texts which are integral to narrative inquiry: "the
use of expressive, contextualized, and vernacular forms of language; the
promotion of emphatic understanding of the lives of characters; and the
creation of a virtual reality" (p. 5). The issue of *virtual reality* is critical
to the practice of narrative inquiry, including how this type of research
is evaluated within the academic community and how resulting texts are
"read" by intended audiences. As Kim notes, "reader identification" is
crucial to the assessment and effectiveness of these texts. The construction of "virtual reality" refers to the reader's ability to "believe in the possibility or the credibility of the virtual world as an analogue to the 'real'
one. Virtual reality is an important element of an arts-based text as it promotes emphatic understanding of the lives of the protagonists" (p. 5).

Narrative Analysis

When using the narrative method, data are analyzed using "narrative
analysis" or "narrative configuration" (Kim, 2006, p. 4). Kim (2006)
explains that *narrative analysis* is a process whereby "the researcher
extracts an emerging theme from the fullness of lived experiences presented in the data themselves and configures stories making a range of
disconnected research elements coherent, so that the story can appeal to
the reader's understanding and imagination" (p. 5).

Researchers employ narrative inquiry in a variety of ways, by asking
a host of research questions. Clandinin and Rosiek (2007) note that narrative inquiry generally focuses on *experience*, which can be conceptualized in numerous ways. Some researchers use this method in order to
access and (re)present various subject positions on a particular topic.
The narrative method is influenced by Bakhtin's theoretical framework.
Bakhtin (1975/1981) compares the narratives of "epics" to those of "novels," asserting that in the epic genre one viewpoint is articulated, whereas
in novels different vantage points are expressed. Researchers influenced
by this framework have developed methods of narrative inquiry aimed at

accessing and (re)presenting multiple viewpoints. An excellent example of this comes from Kim's (2006) work in the field of educational studies.

Kim (2006) applies Bakhtin's framework to narrative inquiry and uses multiple voices positing that individuals with different standpoints (occupying varying positions of power) can help readers to try and understand each participant's viewpoint. Kim conducted research on the viewpoints of people in alternative high schools, from students to administrators. The multimethod research included ethnography, semi-structured interviews with open-ended questions, and narrative inquiry. Kim's work resulted in an arts-based text consisting of five different voices—that is, narratives. The methodology used created a meaningful understanding of the different perspectives operating at this specific site. However, when using this method, the perspectives do not necessarily all take on "relativity," with none being more legitimate or compelling than the others. For example, in Kim's research the narratives were followed by a section called "Epilogue: The Voice of the Researcher," in which a fable was relayed, clearly meant to impart meaning and assist the reader in weighing the various narratives or perspectives. In this way, researchers employing this method can bring a literature review as well as their reflections into the text. In conclusion, Kim suggests that this method is useful for "interrogating the nature of dominant stories" (p. 11), which can be applied to many kinds of research projects and within various critical theoretical frameworks.

Narrative inquiry is increasingly employed as a methodological approach to trauma studies. Trauma studies constitute an expansive and interdisciplinary field and may involve work on the process of trauma and recovery. Harvey, Mishler, Koenan, and Harney (2000) suggest that the narrative approach has led to many new social research questions. They cite examples of narrative research within medical sociology and anthropology that focus on "illness narratives," "suffering narratives," "narratives of hope," and "chronic illness narratives." They also cite a range of studies employing narrative inquiry that focus on the experiences of Holocaust survivors, Vietnam vets, victims of war-related violence, rape survivors, sexual abuse survivors, and African American men's stories of racism.

As many researchers who turn to arts-based practices do, Harvey and colleagues (2000) came to narrative inquiry in their study of sexual trauma survivors when other more traditional research methods failed to fully access the data they were interested in. Their multimethod approach first entailed highly structured interviews used for creating quantitative instruments. Next the team conducted unstructured interviews. Finally the researchers developed a narrative approach, which led to the asking of new research questions. Primarily, these researchers were interested in how survivors (re)make meaning throughout their recovery process (p. 292). Moreover, they were interested in the role and function of survivors' stories in the recovery process (p. 292). The turn to narrative inquiry led them to an array of emergent research questions that can easily be adapted to various research projects.

> How do trauma survivors deal with the problem of constructing a coherent life story and how does the content and form of the story change over time? Do these changes reflect normal developmental processes of trauma recovery? What initiates the restorying of a survivor's narrative and does this have a reparative effect, helping to repair the distorting impact of sexual abuse on normal identity development? What is the relationship between these personal narratives and cultural "master narratives" about women, sexual violence, trauma, and gender identity? How do our expectations and preferences, as clinicians and researchers, for a coherent story interfere with our being able to hear what survivors are trying to tell us? Finally, how can we develop ways of listening to their stories that respect their evolving understandings and their efforts to make meaning of their experiences of sexual trauma? (p. 292)

Based on their research, Harvey and colleagues (2000) identify three major components of narratives: coherence, turning points, and replotting.

The concept of *coherence* refers to how a narrative is communicated. Often there is an assumption that research participants share cohesive narratives; however, particular kinds of survivors may not tell their experiences as "coherent" narratives, which can actually make the narratives more difficult to listen to (Harvey et al., 2000, p. 295). For example, Holocaust survivors may not recount their narrative chronologically as a part of their life story because the depth of the horror is so potent that for them the event "stands outside of time" (Harvey et al., p. 294). Women who have killed their partners as a result of battered woman's syndrome often tell their stories differently over time. Usually initial narratives are not told chronologically as a result of the severe trauma experienced. This has been used against many women during police interviews and court proceedings when police and prosecutors fail to realize that, although initial stories are not relayed cohesively, a restoried and cohesive narrative may later emerge. Researchers need to pay attention to how narratives are communicated—such as talking style, tense, inflection, and tone—which also signal a range of data.

Turning points are often vital to participants' structuring of their narratives and the experiences to which they attest. For example, a turning point may represent a time when the participant went from a victim mindset to a survivor mindset, or might represent another kind of shift in experience or interpretation.

Replotting, or *restorying*, is a primary aspect of narrative research. This is a process whereby participants narrativize their stories through the interplay between cultural frames (available) and individual meaning (which changes over time) (Harvey et al., 2000, p. 307). In addition, restorying is a process that occurs over time as participants reflect on their own major life experiences and reframe them. Replotting can be thought of in the following way: "Since stories express the dialectic between character and plot, in their 'replottings' our respondents position themselves differently than they had in their relationships with significant figures in their lives" (p. 298). Harvey and colleagues (2000) conclude that, in their research, participants engage in restorying to alter the relationship of the past trauma to the present and for the future (p. 301).

Moving beyond a general discussion I review two specific methodological approaches to narrative inquiry that utilize data collected from participants: "biographic narrative interpretive method" and "ghost writing."

Biographical Narrative Interpretive Method

Kip Jones has been at the forefront of advancing narrative inquiry and arts-based research more generally. As a scholar who attended art school, Jones understands key similarities between scientific and artistic practice and, as reviewed in Chapter 1, sees a blurring of the lines between natural science and social science, and scientific inquiry and artistic inquiry. It is within this context that Jones developed a "visual perspective" on qualitative interviews. Jones draws on his fine-arts training in order to consider the visual aspects of qualitative interview. His major contribution in this area is in identifying the ways in which the qualitative interview process, from data collection to analysis and write-up, are *already* visual processes and thus better attune researchers to these aspects of their practices.

Theoretically this methodological practice is influenced by Bakhtin's work that posits the centrality of the border of the "verbal and nonverbal." Using this framework Jones creates a set of practices at the intersection of a *visual perspective* and *narrative perspective* onto the interview method. He argues that all qualitative researchers engage in a visualiza-

tion process as they assemble their participants' stories, "creatively building a story" with sets of "visual impressions" (2001, p. 3). Jones writes:
"The bricolage of images and nonverbal clues accumulated to produce
additional keys that unlocked the narratives, enriched the life stories and
enhanced the analyses" (p. 3).

Additionally, Jones draws on his art school background regarding
the negative space that surrounds and thus gives presence to a positive
object (a basic point of fact in the discipline of fine art). He explains
that in interviews negative space also surrounds or frames dialogue. He
notes, "I have tried to further develop my visual skills in my narrative biographical work. One of the tricks is, I believe, to work on seeing better
in order to get a better picture of the people whom we encounter in our
research" (2001, p. 2).

It was only after developing a visual perspective in his social research
that Jones "began to see attempts at verbal description as a device that storytellers used to express the physical, the sensual and the atmospheric"
(2001, p. 5). These dimensions of social life, and our encounters with
them via ethnographic observations and interviews, are largely impen-
etrable by traditional research methods. Yet it is within and across these
dimensions that the soul of our participants' experiences may emerge.
In this vein, the materialization of innovative arts-based forms of narrative research respond to long-standing objectives guiding qualitative
research—getting at *real*, textured, complex, sensory, contextual meanings.

It is within the context of these understandings that Jones employs a
biographical narrative interpretive method. This method relies on a *minimalist passive interviewing technique,* in which the researchers engage in an
ongoing interpretive process. A minimalist passive interview technique
refers to an interview situation where "noninterruption" is practiced
(Jones, 2003, p. 62). For example, a researcher begins with one open,
"narrative-inducing" question and then proceeds to allow the participant
to tell his or her story without interruption (p. 61). Rapport is maintained via appropriate visual cues such as eye contact and nodding. This
method of interview is based on the idea that preconceived questions or
even broad lines of inquiry may obscure parts of potential data that are
"nested" within something else (p. 61). After the initial noninterruption
interview, generally lasting 45–60 minutes, a process of analysis occurs.
Then a second interview session where follow-up questions are asked
occurs, followed again by analysis and, depending on the need, a third
interview session.

Jones identifies gestalt as a central theoretical principle of working
with this method. He defines *gestalt* as "the constructed shape of a story,

through theme, motif and/or various agendas—hidden or otherwise" (2003, p. 62). By using an interview technique of noninterruption the gestalt of the participant's story retains its integrity.

Each interview session is transcribed verbatim, with researcher notes. Jones finds the note-taking process central to building metaphors and gaining understanding of key issues. There are various kinds of memo notes a researcher may find helpful. For example, "on-the-fly" notes may consist of key words or phrases (Hesse-Biber & Leavy, 2006b, p. 258). "Personal matters and reflexivity notes" are a space where the researcher takes notes about his or her feelings, concerns, shifting position within the project, and so forth (Hesse-Biber & Leavy, 2006b, p. 259). In addition to standard descriptive field notes and ongoing data analysis notes, these kinds of memo-taking practices may be particularly useful when using this method.

Jones also employs *reflective teams* for analysis. The team analysis approach focuses on two dimensions of the data: the "lived life" and the "told story" (2003, p. 62). The use of analysis teams coupled with the different analysis poles helps to ensure scientific standards designed to suit this method. Jones writes: "Objectivity is maintained by keeping each stage of the analysis discrete as well as involving different teams of researchers in a process of hypothesizing and developing themes" (p. 62). In this vein, a microanalysis of the lived life and a thematic analysis of the told story occurs. Jones notes:

> Biographical details and themes are tested against in-depth analysis of the text, examining hesitancy, repetition, contradictions and pauses. Through hypothesizing how the lived life informs the told story, the case history is then finally constructed from the two separate threads of the "lived story" and the "told story." A case structure is then formulated that validates more than one event based upon the actions of the interviewee. (p. 63)

In general narrative researchers, regardless of their specific methodology, can gain trustworthiness by making their research purpose transparent and then "set[ting] what they deem to be the appropriate context for storying the data" (Clandinin & Connelly, 1989, p. 19).

Jones developed this method in order to access "essence," which may be flattened or rendered invisible by traditional interview practices. Moreover, Jones draws on Law and Urry (2004) and suggests that traditional methods are not able to reveal the "sensory," "emotional," and "kinaesthetic." Therefore, he advocates a rigorous method of biographical narrative interview as a way of getting at contextual, sensual, and kinaesthetic knowledge (2006, p. 3).

Ghostwriting and Narrative

Carl Rhodes (2000) provides researchers with a new way to conceptualize their place within the knowledge-building process and eventual textual representation. In everyday language, *ghostwriters* are understood to be writers who are commissioned to author the stories attributed to others, a common tool used by celebrities, for example, who foray into writing memoirs. Rhodes adopts the term as a metaphor for how researchers can understand their role within the production of textual representations of the data they collect from research subjects.

With respect to traditional qualitative writing Rhodes asserts, "I am, therefore, in the text, but rather than being explicit, I am hidden; I am like a ghost" (2000, p. 511). As storytellers, social researchers are in fact collaborators and co-creators of knowledge with research participants, whether in oral histories, in-depth interviews, or ethnography. The metaphor of ghostwriting extends beyond a new term to account for the position of the researcher within the text by offering a critique of traditional transcription and related strategies connected to representation. Two interconnected issues are paramount: *reflexivity* and *voice*. Rhodes argues that the traditional model for writing up interview results, for example, actually obscures the role of the researcher in the process, thus making reflexivity and transparency all the more difficult to achieve. Specifically Rhodes explains that conventional qualitative writing often relies on quoted transcript excerpts or entire transcripts that may appear as appendices. This format implies that the text is a "representation" of what the informant or informants have said and may consequently render invisible the role of the researcher in *eliciting that information*, from scheduling the interview, to asking guiding questions, to selecting quotes for the written report.

As an alternative to these standard transcription practices, Rhodes (2000) engages in an intensely personal yet systematic and rigorous process of turning his interviews into narratives—that is, into coherent stories. This exemplifies the issue of coherence reviewed earlier, although in this case Rhodes is after coherent narratives.

Here, the motivation for developing an arts-based method is a direct result of theoretical and epistemological concerns. Put differently, while feminist and critical theoretical insights shine a light on the subjective and situated aspects of research, Rhodes delineates a methodological plan for actively using these insights in the execution of narrative research. In the following excerpt he details part of the process of how he went about writing the story of one informant whom he calls "Bob." As a point of information, Bob told his story episodically, and thus Rhodes had to "regenre" it in order to produce a linear tale. As noted throughout this chapter, other researchers refer to this process as "restorying," which allows the researcher to analyze stories for key elements and then represent them chronologically in order to provide causal links and thus create meaning (Ollerenshaw & Creswell, 2002). At the point we enter the excerpt, Rhodes has already done some initial interpretive work and determined the particular narrative structure he would follow.

> Next I read back through my notes to ensure that the overall structure that I had developed from memory was consistent with what I had written down in the interview. From there, I started the actual writing. Based on narrative ordering that I had developed earlier, I went through my notes and started typing out the story. I would skip back and forth through my notes, reordering the flow of conversation to follow the plot line of the written story. In doing so, I incorporated as many direct quotations and turns of phrase that Bob had used as possible, and worked to tell the story in a similar tenor to what he had used in conversation. After going through and rewriting my entire interview notes in this way, I read through the text a number of times, checking and making changes to ensure that the story developed in line with my chosen narrative structure, that the character development occurred in line with the plot of the story, and that the story line effectively built through to a tension between the main characters. Again, despite my intervention, my intent was to retain the characters, themes, plot, and setting from the interview conversation but to reorder them into the format of a written narrative similar to that of an autobiography. This written story, however, was not intended to be a replica of the interview but was designed to create a written narrative congruent in feel and content to the discussion that transpired in the interview. The text was then returned to Bob for review and feedback; all of his recommended modifications were subsequently incorporated into the text. This process of review and rewriting was iterated three times. ... (2000, pp. 517–518)

As you can see from this example, Rhodes engaged in a systematic and multitiered interpretation and writing process drawing on some of the tenets of grounded theory, sharing authority, and literary narrative. Furthermore, the ghostwriting approach to constructing Bob's story required continuous reflexivity. Although the elimination of traditional transcription may at first glance appear to place more creative control with the researcher, in fact, as Rhodes suggests, it is this very practice of ghostwriting that allows the researcher to account for his or her position in the textual production, as opposed to disavowing it or glossing over it, even if unintentionally. This methodology results in a story that is derived directly from the data collected and also shaped in collaboration with research participants. In this respect, this strategy is attentive to questions of "voice" and what Skinner (2003) refers to as "the ethics of writing," meaning the balance found between the writer's voice and the voices of the participants (p. 527). In short, this method merges co-created data with several tenets of autobiographical work in a highly reflexive and collaborative context.

- How does the rise in autobiographical data challenge the public–private dichotomy?
- What are the different strategies available for researchers to explicitly incorporate their subjectivity into their stories?
- How do researchers use autobiographical data? What are the rewards and challenges of writing about oneself?

The Rise of Autobiographical Input

Alhough historically even qualitative researchers such as ethnographers were charged with rendering "objective" accounts of social reality, it is now well accepted that ethnographers are positioned within the texts they produce. In fact, ethnographers communicate partial and situated realities while they also become constituent parts of those represented realities. In other words, although traditionally presenting themselves as "invisible" within their texts, ethnographers, like all social researchers, are implicitly interwoven into their final representations in many ways.

Moreover, autobiographical writing is often intermingled with representations of other persons or groups. In the case of ethnography—for example, field notes, on-the-fly notes, memo notes—theoretical memos and analysis memos require the researcher to write his or her understandings and impressions of a particular social reality. This includes the assumptions the researcher brings to bear on how he or she views the world as well as his or her particular experiences in that reality (which include emotional, psychological, physical, intellectual, and practical field experiences). Therefore, for ethnographers, engaging with questions of reflexivity not only requires attention to how standpoint and power shape perception, but also how to communicate an experience while living it (Skinner, 2003, p. 527). The "thick descriptions" that result from this process are therefore informed not by the researcher's neutral rendering of events, but rather by his or her subjective experience in that reality, and in the best of cases, by his or her systematic reflexivity about the experience.

Furthermore, as researchers try to weave their experiences into a coherent narrative that can be distributed to an audience, most engage in a process similar to practices of literary narrative. In this respect, some researchers merely draw on literary conceptions of storytelling while, as reviewed later, others actually draw on elements of fiction as well (to varying degrees).

In Chapter 1 I reviewed the major dualisms that traditionally guided the practice of social research as well as the challenges to the subject–object and rational–emotional dichotomies posed by scholars in the qualitative paradigm. The explicit use of the researcher as the subject of inquiry challenges yet another long-standing dichotomy: the public–private split. It is for this reason that opposition to autobiographical work can at times be strong. Autobiographical social research rejects the public–private dichotomy, exposing it as a false dualism, and suggests that the private is indeed public, and vice versa. For this and other reasons the use of "the personal" in social research is both contested and complex; however, it is the contention of most qualitative practitioners that the personal is always, to some extent, embedded within research practice and resulting knowledge.

As stated earlier, traditional ethnography requires an ongoing subjective writing and interpretation process, and in recent years ethnographers have only become more reflexive about this process. Likewise, feminist researchers have persuasively demonstrated how false claims of neutrality mask and perpetuate the construction of gendered, racialized, sexed, and classed knowledge (see Halpin, 1989; Smith, 1987). It is in this context that Sandra Harding (1993) proposed "strong objectivity"—attention to the context of discovery and not just the context of justification—as a means of reflexively situating oneself in his or her research. Moreover, Freeman (2007) suggests that autobiography is necessarily a form of narrative inquiry. With this said, here I consider *autoethnography* as a wide-ranging method of self-study.

Autoethnographic Narratives

Autoethnography is a method of self-study in which the researcher is viewed as a viable data source. Autoethnographic writing is distinct. Ellis (2004) notes, "*Autoethnography* refers to writing about the personal and its relationship to culture. It is an autobiographical genre of writing and research that displays multiple layers of consciousness" (p. 37, quoting Dumont, 1978, original emphasis). Pelias (2004) suggests the purpose of autoethnographic writing is *resonance* (p. 11). As with all arts-based research, this kind of writing creates "me too" moments for readers (Pelias, 2004). Moreover, this method accesses the "nexus of self and culture" using the "self as a springboard, as a witness" (p. 11).

The recent rise in autoethnography as a stand-alone method, or as a tool used in multimethod research projects, is linked to a surge in academic literature about the role of the researcher in the research process and the overall increase in qualitative sociology. In this respect, autoethnography has become more popular, partly as a result of the theoretical and epistemological challenges to traditional positivism posed by feminism, postmodernism, poststructuralism, multiculturalism, cultural studies, and general increases in interdisciplinary research. As researchers working from critical perspectives such as feminism have challenged the subject–object, rational–emotional, and concrete–abstract dualisms that have historically guided social scientific inquiry, a space has opened for researchers to create methods and methodologies that not only account for a researcher's subjectivity but also refashion the researcher as the primary subject of investigation (or one of several overlapping sources of data). The most common of these methodological innovations is *autoethnography*, which is often communicated through stories or narratives.

Impressionistic autoethnography is an emergent method that is generally used in ethnographic research, thereby merging data about others and self. Skinner, a social anthropologist at the forefront of research with and about this method, draws on the work of Van Maanen (1988) and defines it as follows:

> Impressionistic ethnography is a blend of inside-out writing with an Impressionist's representational style (figurative, personalized, fleeting, dramatic and part realist/confessional). ... This writing begins with the self, with embedding the self before engaging relationally with the other. The intention is to paint a composite picture based upon a consistency of fieldwork days. ... I would argue that this epistemologically justifiable mode of research writing does not go too far, but does go some way towards overcoming the problem of self—quite literally self denial—in the social sciences. (2003, p. 514)

This new approach to merging ethnographic and autobiographical data is an important development in this field; however, in this book I focus primarily on *narrative autoethnography*, which is traditional autoethnographic writing that is represented as a narrative or story.

Narrative autoethnography exists on a continuum beginning with researchers sharing personal experiences with their respondents, which then become part of the larger research narrative, to wholly autobiographical projects, to those that explicitly combine autobiographical data and fiction. Let's first consider autoethnography as an extension of ethnographic research.

Ethnography has come to be understood as a deeply personal research experience (Van Maanen, 1988). As noted, over the past several decades ethnographers have started to write increasingly personal accounts of their experiences in the field as opposed to attempts at presenting the neutral-observer stance prevalent in earlier publications. As a result, some researchers have come to see autoethnography as an extension of what ethnographers already do (Berger, 2001) and thus use narrative autoethnography as a part of larger ethnographic research projects. In this design researchers share their experiences as a part of their ethnographic work—as a means of developing their own ideas, questioning their assumptions and positionality, building rapport, and creating reciprocity. Coffey (1999) explains that ethnographers negotiate and write their identities during the research process. With this in mind, autoethnography can also assist the researcher in this identity work (although Coffey is concerned that autoethnography can become self-indulgent and sacrifice rigor).

Leigh Berger (2001) used narrative autoethnography as a part of ethnographic work done with a religious group called Dalet Shalom Messianic Congregation, a group that maintains cultural ties to Judaism and a belief that Jesus is the Messiah. The incorporation of her own personal stories was vital to her research for two main reasons. First, through sharing her stories, ideas, and beliefs with her research participants, Berger was able to develop and maintain the rapport that is integral to field research. Moreover, with highly sensitive subject matter such as religion and spirituality, gaining trust, building rapport, and indeed making oneself vulnerable becomes essential to the process. In this respect, elements of autoethnography can be employed as a strategy for eliciting data from research participants. Second, as researchers who deal with delicate subject matter or those engaged in robust qualitative research often find, Berger's feelings, ideas, and beliefs were surfacing, developing, and *transforming* as she experienced a range of emotional and intellectual challenges. This kind of research requires high levels of reflexivity and openness on the part of the researcher throughout the process, as well as an ability and willingness to interpret the data through different lenses. Berger achieved all of this through the narrative autoethnographic aspect of the research design. Berger writes, "Thinking, writing, and rewriting all lead me to new understandings of my experiences" (p. 507). She goes on to explain how this method allowed her to "access new perceptions and worldviews" (p. 509) that would have otherwise remained untapped. This is an example of how an arts-based approach is chosen in order to meet research objectives—in this case, fostering the high levels of rapport and reflexivity needed to effectively complete the data-sensitive study.

As noted earlier, some researchers perform narrative autoethnography as a stand-alone method. Carolyn Ellis has been at the forefront of advancing autoethnographic research and defines this method as follows:

> "What is autoethnography?" you might ask. My brief answer: research, writing, story, and method that connect the autobiographical and personal to the cultural, social, and political. Autoethnographic forms feature concrete action, emotion, embodiment, self-consciousness, and introspection portrayed in dialogue, scenes, characterization, and plot. Thus, autoethnography claims the conventions of literary writing. (2004, p. xix)

This method combines autobiographical writing with the conventions of narrative writing, often incorporating fiction (although certainly not always). Autoethnography may be communicated as a short story, essay, poem, novel, play, performance piece, or other experimental text. Researchers often fictionalize aspects of the work in order to create characterizations (which may be composites), as a means of situating the piece within a particular cultural and historical context, to evoke mood or emotionality, or to follow plot conventions. In autoethnographic writing, fiction is therefore employed as a means of emphasizing particular partial truths, revealing social meanings, and linking the experiences of individuals to the larger cultural and institutional context in which social actors live. In this respect, this form of experimental writing can help qualitative researchers *bridge the micro and macro levels of analysis* and accentuate particular aspects of their work (such as subjugated voices).

A primary advantage of this method is the possibility it has to *raise self-consciousness* and thereby *promote reflexivity*. However, placing oneself at the center of the research process carries its own set of considerations and burdens. Autoethnography requires the researcher to make him- or herself vulnerable. One cannot predict the emotions one will experience throughout this process. In addition, by opening up his or her personal life to the public, a researcher lets go of some privacies and invites possible criticism. In this respect, some think of autoethnography as "writing on the edge—and without a safety net" (Vickers, 2002, p. 608). This can be painful. For this reason, as well as a measure towards validity, it is important to have a support team in place to offer feedback throughout the process (Tenni, Smyth, & Boucher, 2003).

- Why use narrative autoethnography? What kinds of
  research questions can be addressed with this method?

Autoethnographic research can be used to address a number of research questions, including those linked to exploring personal or shared traumas; the grieving process; spirituality; the life cycle, or major life markers such as partnering, uncoupling, pregnancy, and parenting; or topics such as organizational life, illness, stigmas, oppression, and subjugation; and many other issues.

Margaret H. Vickers (2002) used narrative autoethnography to explore both her experience of grief (over her degenerative illness as well as her husband's) as well as the severe abuse she dealt with in her workplace (also related to her illness). In her short stories, Vickers explores her feelings and experiences surrounding her multiple sclerosis, as well as the depression she suffers from, and simultaneous feelings of loss and grief pertaining to her husband's illness (a chronic lung condition that spread to his brain, affecting his abilities and personality and forcing him to retire at the age of 43)—she writes that she feels he has already died.

Vickers's (2002) haunting work offers alternative ways of conceptualizing the sick–well dichotomy as well as communicating profound feelings of loss, fear, and despair that, in her words, make her life now only about "existing," that "there is nothing to look forward to" (p. 611), and that things will only worsen. Vickers is also able to explore the oppression she faced at work as well as her coping strategies for dealing with it, along with her other significant life challenges. The autobiographical story form evokes emotion for the reader and allows for a cathartic release. The following is a brief excerpt.

> The dark hood of melancholy once again envelops me—slowing me; constraining me; bringing unimaginable loneliness. As I consider my life, I feel hollow, empty, numb ... I exist now. I do not enjoy, rarely feel anything but hollow, emptiness. I record another day of unhappiness; another spoke in the wheel carrying me down, but where? ... I cry a lot. My thoughts are interrupted and the tears hastily brushed away. I take the phone call from one of the intermediaries from the study: Shelly is not doing very well. ... Michael thinks the tears are for her. The tears are for me; for my pain, my fear, my loss. Not *hers*, not *his*—mine! (p. 613)

This autobiographical method of story-writing is critical, in this example, for creating new knowledge about the *experience* of pain, loss, grief, and illness. Differing from other methods, the autoethnographic short story allows the emotional experience to be conveyed as a part of the knowledge itself; the writing is not sterile, and is actually even difficult to read. This is critical. The researcher is also allowed to explore her feelings and experiences, thus validating her experiences as legitimate data that are just as valid as those of others she might choose to study. Moreover, this approach broadens traditional qualitative understandings of "insider status" (Vickers, 2002, p. 609) by positioning the researcher as both informant and writer. Therefore, this method also problematizes the *insider–outsider dichotomy* that guides traditional qualitative research practice. In this regard, it is important to note that the method revolves around writing—the written word—more so than traditional qualitative methods such as interviewing and field research, which rely heavily on verbal communication and visual observations. In the case of autoethnographic narratives the researcher is writing, not speaking—an entirely different process (for example, most people can speak more quickly than they can write) (Hesse-Biber & Leavy, 2006b; Maines, 2001, p. 109).

Other researchers have similarly used this method as a way of exploring grief, but with the express intent of creating connections with others. For example, Jonathan Wyatt (2005) wrote an (auto)ethnographic short story about his father's death. In writing about his father's last days, death, and funeral, his narrative also explores key issues of family, loss, and the father–son relationship. Communicated as a performance piece (with the intent to publish it later as a short story), Wyatt shared the narrative as a means of creating human connection with audience members and exploring, with others, central aspects of the human condition. The story format also allowed Wyatt to experiment with issues of time as opposed to presenting a linear account, as is often the case in academic writing.

Shamla McLaurin (2003) used the autoethnographic short story format to work through her struggle with homophobia, which, through this format, she was able to situate within the context of her own biography as it is lived within a larger social context. As she chronicled her struggles with homophobia McLaurin also raised complex issues pertaining to race, gender, religious ideology, and family beliefs, all entwined in the various homophobic messages she had received throughout her life. Similarly, Sarah N. Gatson (2003) used this method in order to explore racial identity, making key links between her personal multiracial identity issues and the context of racial identity in the United States. Ronald J. Pelias (2003, p. 369) has used this method to critically examine the academy; the autoethnographic story format has allowed him to construct "a sociology of the academy."

The Use of Fiction in Social Research

Fiction is one lens or tool that can be used to shape narrative inquiry. When thinking about the use of fiction in anthropology, Katherine Frank (2000) poses the following questions:

> Could fiction be a partial answer to some of the political problems of attempting objective representation? When should an anthropologist or researcher tell ethnographically informed short stories? More important, what can an anthropologist accomplish using fiction, and what is given up in the process? These questions may have no final answers; rather, they can serve as an entrée into open-ended discussions about truth, representation and audience. (p. 482)

As discussed, the elements of narrative, fiction, and autobiography can make their way into research projects in many different ways, spanning a continuum from mostly "found" or "co-created" data, to that which is largely fictionalized, or communicated via the tools of literary fiction. Fictionalized short stories are generally thought of as the *representation* stage of research; however, fiction can be expressly used as both a part of *narrative practice* as well as the *form* representation takes. Experimental ethnographers have been at the forefront of using fiction as a mode of practice and a representational vehicle.

- When is it appropriate for narrative researchers to use fiction?
- How can fiction aid the interpretive process?
- Who is the audience for ethnographic fiction? How does fiction communicate with its audience?
- How can fiction be employed in the service of social justice issues, such as feminist concerns or the study of power on micro and macro levels?

Frank (2000) advocates considering fiction as a part of research design when "factual representation obscures possible alternative interpretations" (p. 482). In other words, as researchers who challenge positivist principles understand, traditional representational forms that typically result in an account or finite set of conclusions may render invisible those interpretations not put forth by the researcher, creating the false appearance of a "truth" that has been "discovered." Fiction can, ironically, expose that which "factual representation" conceals by its very implication. In addition, fiction may reach broader audiences and do so on deeper levels as compared with other forms of academic writing. In this regard, Diversi (1998) explains, "the short story genre has the potential to render lived experience with more verisimilitude than does the traditional realist text, for it enables the reader to feel that interpretation is never finished or complete" (p. 132).

Fiction also presents an opportunity for those interested in contributing to public sociology or public anthropology. This writing format allows social science research to (potentially) reach broader audiences than the highly specialized academic audiences that usually benefit from ethnographic research (Diversi, 1998), because it does not rely on academic jargon, circulates more widely, and may be more engaging to a broader range of readers (Frank, 2000).

Some ethnographers turn to fiction as a means of working through or restructuring their ideas. In this vein, Frank explains that she turns to fiction when she is not sure where to place her ideas or findings in relation to existing academic literature (p. 486). For instance, by placing her work within an existing literature, it can become limited, with possible alternative theoretical engagement or interpretations blocked.

For example, I turned to experimental writing when I was engaged in a historical sociology project investigating how journalists and other groups have represented selected historical events over the past century. My primary research method was content analysis of documents, images, films, and so forth. During my research into the representation of the *Titanic* disaster over time, I was struck by a tabloid magazine cover story. The fabricated cover photo depicted a baby girl floating in the ocean with a *Titanic* life preserver, and the caption exclaimed that a *Titanic* survivor had been discovered alive after 80 years! The data ultimately did not fit into my research design; however, I found myself thinking about them.

Through the process of pondering the photograph and headline I was able to flesh out loose associations that were deep under the surface of my data. I was conducting a thematic content analysis, and one of the themes to emerge focused on the meanings the *Titanic* has been imbued with over time. For example, the sinking of the *Titanic* has been conceptualized by some as a "turning point" in Western society, representing the end of one kind of society and the metaphoric beginning of modern technological–capitalist society. I intently considered the stereotypical representations of immigrants who were traveling from Europe to the United States on the *Titanic*, and I began to think about metaphorical points of convergence between that journey and the earlier European explorers/settlers and the violence they visited upon the Native Americans. All of these musings were not a part of my formal research project; however, I used a fictional experimental writing form to "work through" these issues. The resulting piece, entitled "Fish Soup," was not published as a part of the book in which this research is embedded, but it did clarify my thinking and was a part of one final version of the work. Moreover, this process aided how I theoretically conceptualized the found images and documents that *were* a primary part of my research methodology. In this regard, although the resulting writing itself was not formally a part of my research project, the process of writing the piece aided the continued theoretical refinement of key issues of representation central to my work.

FISH SOUP (2007)

Floating in the cascading tears of the Atlantic for over eighty years I remain unchainged. Cryogenically frozen, moving. Bodies that do not succumb to Time. An eighty year old infant girl waiting for her mother's swollen breast. I have waited. Floating. The character through which so many caricatures have been resErected. I am the origin of representations. Follow the point. I am the sound of a hand smacking the fleshless face of simulation–imitation. And now/ my silences **scream.**

Their sinking chorus can rest. Through kNEW light seeping, old shadows fall sleepy—sleepy I/eyes, as ghosts are allowed to haunt in cameralight. In the zone, the celebrity ozone.

Over eighty years—an infant baby girl for over, those years. WithOUT words of a lasting language eye share our histories. Truthful accounts of fictions told through simulated re/collections. This wAS the night as I re-member it. Remembered memories. Harmony undone. Self discovered to un ravel.

The crash made us hear/here what glossed our resin but eluded discernible vision. Cold. So damn cold in hear. The ice *was* fallen. Before WE knew of the collision, the knowing knowers k(new) the un/knowable. My haunted memory shadows me. And haunts realized, necessitated, NO, Demanded manifestation. Death in festival. A CARNivAL end. Now they have their/history. I/eye *have* history my haunted memory. Again, CONsumption.

Bodies attached to callused hands that writhe. We are coming. Mother. MATTER. My mother must have been quite wealthy as they are still searching for me. No. It must have been my father. Squash snakes. Applesauce. New systems ceiling fates they imprison their own. Selling our buying beaten body(s). Wanting to make my history—for it to envelop you. A dreaming slumber. The playful dead are not altogether powerless you know.

Fish Soup. Come. Come on. Your child's heart beats to our chorus. Their hearts, our pace. Makers. Rewrite what is all done. Come undone. I, an eighty year old infant baby boygirl come undone. (W)rite me repeatedly. (W)rite me. I see you coming. The unfamiliar pierce of a safety ships' rescue light. A flag. I am a thread unraveling within it. I see you, you come. Picture taking killing boxes hanging from hung necks. Come. Come (un)save me. I shall be still. Very still. An UNknowing

infant baby girl without language(s). Come steal an image-mirage. Find your fallen
angel. Ascendancy. Bright light/Brighter. Come on. I will be very, very still.

Fiction also allows the researcher to reexamine his or her findings
in a new context which can lead to a refinement or elaboration of theoretical and other insights. In this way, Frank insightfully identifies fiction
as a problem-solving strategy (2000, p. 485).

In terms of practice, fiction can also be employed as a part of a
methodology that is consistent with feminist, postmodern, postcolonial, or other critical perspectives on social power. This methodological
device has developed in the context of new theoretical perspectives on
power, and thus serves as an example of how theory drives methodological innovation.

An excellent example comes from Frank's (2000) work. In this study
Frank engaged in multitiered participant observation in the sex industry,
observing, systematically interviewing, and herself working in five different kinds of strip clubs (thus taking on the role of participant). She
then wrote an ethnographically informed fictional narrative called "The
Management of Hunger," in which she created composite characters
informed by her experiences and the people from the settings, as well
as her own ideas about them. By using fiction Frank was able to describe
the nuances of the setting and constituent relationships in complex and
detailed ways to an audience who may not already be familiar with that
kind of environment. Furthermore, she was able to access the complexity of the power relations enacted through the relationships in the field
without flattening them to the one-dimensional relations of "oppression" or "seduction" espoused in much of the academic literature on sex
work. Frank reflects on her research as follows:

> My own experiences as both a sex worker and as an ethnographer of sex
> workers and their customers suggest that sex work involves moments of
> empowerment, intimacy, and gratification alongside moments of degrada-
> tion, alienation, or disenchantment—it is this amalgamation of power and
> pleasure that I explore in my fiction. There is a possibility of portraying a
> complexity of lived experience in fiction that might not always come across
> in a theoretical explication, even one that is concerned with elucidating the
> complexity of power relations and human interactions. (p. 483)

Frank's work suggests that the texture of human experience, partly
informed by the complex relationship between the structural contexts
in which we operate and our own agency, can be accessed and expressed
via the tools of fiction. For this reason, this approach to research may

be particularly appealing to critical scholars engaged in feminist, queer studies, postcolonial, or multicultural research.

An extension of this thinking suggests that fiction can also help feminist and other researchers bridge the divide often felt as we try to attend to the voices of our research participants as well as to our own feminist or critical theoretical commitments. For example, in power-rich environments like the sex industry, in which gender and sexual identity are dominant categories of experience, researchers may find a disjuncture between what their respondents say, what they observe, and what the literature claims. Fiction can be a mode for accounting for these disjunctures, perceptions, and perspectives of the social reality, providing a way for accentuating the many overlapping layers of human experience. In addition, as feminist researchers often note, there can be difficulty when trying to account both for the voices of our research participants and our own theoretical commitments to feminist principles and to the larger project of feminism of which our work is a part (Leavy, 2007). Particularly for feminists, the challenge is often to account for how our research participants are discursively constituted subjects while also giving voice to their perspectives and experiences (Saukko, 2000). Fiction can be a medium in which feminist researchers can reconcile some of these conflicts and find ways of writing both the knowledge their subjects share with them and their insights into how larger contexts and systems shape their subjects (their attitudes, perceptions, and experiences).

Finally, when thinking about what is meant by fiction and short story writing as a representational form, it helps to consider various categories of writing. Robert E. Rinehart (1998) distinguishes between ethnography, fiction, and fictional ethnography while acknowledging slippage among these categories. Frank adds the category *"creative nonfiction"* to denote "a vivid journalistic style using fictional techniques" (2000, p. 483). The technique I have emphasized is *fictional ethnography* (sometimes called *experimental ethnography*), which merges ethnographic research with fiction, although you can apply these ideas to many different kinds of studies (including intensive interview, oral history, or focus-group research).

Data Analysis and Trustworthiness in Fiction-Based Narrative Research

The strongest critique of autobiographically driven narrative research is that it may not be trustworthy or meet the standards of social scientific knowledge—the knowledge is simply "too subjective." This concern is based on positivist and postpositivist criteria for measuring validity and reliability, which are not appropriate ways of thinking through analysis issues regarding this genre of data. Similar concerns and fears emerge with respect to research that draws explicitly on fiction as a part of practice and/or representation.

Historically, both academic research and public perception have been informed by the *fiction–nonfiction dualism* that inherently legitimizes the notion of a discernible "truth," while implying fiction to be its polar opposite; however, it is now widely accepted in academia that there are "truths" to be found in fiction, and nonfiction also draws on aspects of fiction in its rendering of social reality. In other words, the polarization of "fiction" and "nonfiction" is misleading, and qualitative social science research is moving beyond this false dichotomy.

- How can autobiographical data be analyzed? How can trustworthiness be achieved? How can this kind of data be judged?
- How can ethnographically grounded fiction be authenticated? How is validity conceptualized with respect to fictional writings?
- How can disconnected, nonlinear, or episodic data be transformed into coherent stories, if "coherence" is an aim?
- When analyzing and representing data via the tools of fiction, what are the particular ethical considerations researchers must consider?

There are many strategies available for analyzing qualitative data, including those that are (partly) autobiographical or fictional. Although analysis and interpretation choices should always be congruent with the overall methodological design, epistemological and theoretical viewpoints of the research, and specific research objectives, I will offer some approaches to the analysis and interpretation of autobiographical data as well as data that are obtained ethnographically and later represented in narrative formats.

When working with this genre of data, it is important to begin analysis early in the research process and engage repeatedly in cycles of analysis (Tenni et al., 2003). When researchers use their own experiences as a part of data collection, there may be a tendency to collect too much data, to not know when to stop (Tenni et al., 2003). By analyzing the data in cycles, beginning early in the collection process, researchers are better able to recognize when they have reached "data saturation," which is the point at which the collection of more data stops adding to the insights gained and the researcher risks being inundated (Coffey, 1999).

Researchers using this kind of data must also be in tune to their emotional, carnal, psychological, and intellectual indicators. Traditionally researchers, particularly in the positivist tradition, have been taught to disavow their feelings; however, these kinds of internal signals are vital to building authentic and trustworthy knowledge when using unconventional qualitative methods. Tenni and colleagues (2003) refer to this as engaging in an "internal dialogue" with ourselves. This is especially important in autoethnography or sensitive field research where a researcher may experience discomfort, sadness, or any number of disconcerting feelings (Ellis, 2004; Tenni et al., 2003). Keeping a diary is one strategy for consistently noting where one is located within the process (Tenni et al., 2003).

It is also advisable to engage in an "external dialogue" throughout the data collection and analysis process. This adds two features to the research process. First, there is a built-in support system for the researcher, who, as stated, may experience unexpected emotions during the process. Second, this adds a built-in dimension of validity to the resulting knowledge. As noted earlier, Jones (2006) employs a team approach to analysis toward this end.

- How can theory aid the analysis process?

Tenni and colleagues (2003) also suggest explicitly using theory during data analysis in order to open up the data to new interpretations and alternate meanings. One strategy for using theory is to identify the level of analysis the research is occurring on and then view the data from a theoretical lens on a different level (Tenni et al., 2003). In other words, the researcher views data that operate on the micro level from a macro theoretical perspective, and vice versa. For example, let's take Vickers's autoethnographic research on her illness and the related abuse she experienced in the workplace and apply this data analysis strategy. Vickers's data occurs at the individual level; however, by applying macro theories, perhaps organizational theory, new interpretations of her experience of illness and related abuse in the workplace may surface. Applying a macro perspective such as feminism to her experience of loss during her husband's illness and her need to cry "for herself" may offer new insights onto this profoundly personal experience, placing it in a larger cultural context of gender relations.

- How can the audience determine what is derived from found data and what is communicated via a fictional lens?

Finally, regardless of how researchers inject validity and authenticity into their analysis and writing, they must consider how to represent their methodological strategies. It is critical, when working with the tools of fiction, that researchers be explicit about what aspects of the work are grounded in observations or interviews and what is derived from personal ideas or fantasies (Frank, 2000). Fictionalized narratives derived from a literature review or found documents should also be clearly explained as such. Social researchers who employ fiction need to disclose, for example, when they have created composite characters or conventional plotlines versus when they are creating a characterization based on a particular individual or when they are recounting an experience that specifically occurred. These kinds of disclosures are critical to ethical practice and simultaneously strengthen the trustworthiness of the data.

Checklist of Considerations

When considering using methods of narrative inquiry and contemplating issues of research design, it may be helpful to ask yourself the following:

✓ What are the goals of my study? How does narrative inquiry respond to my research questions? Could other methods address my research questions?

✓ If using autobiographical data, how will I recognize the saturation point in data collection? Will I begin data analysis early in the process? What kind of support team do I have in place, and how will they participate in the analysis and interpretation of data?

✓ How will I use theory? How will I employ theoretical lenses that operate on different levels, as well as those that may differ from my first inclinations?

✓ If using fiction in my writing, who is the audience for my research? How will fiction help illuminate the data? How will I account for my representational choices in ways that are ethical, paying attention to key issues of reflexivity and voice? How will I create trustworthiness?

Conclusion

This chapter has offered an introduction to narrative inquiry. Under the umbrella of "narrative research" there are a host of interview methods reliant on collecting data from participants as well as those that involve self-study. In addition, researchers employ both nonfiction and fiction lenses onto the analysis and writing process. Work done in this area results in representations in many forms, from research articles to poems, short stories, dramatic scripts, and novels. These reflexive writings seek to artistically reveal essence and create a resonance between the writer and reader.

In the following essay Karen Scott-Hoy chronicles her responses to the attacks of September 11, 2001, reflexively examining her reaction to the event as a mother and an Australian citizen. The piece illustrates how narrative autoethnography can be used to explore serious issues, as experienced and perceived by individuals, while placing those issues in a larger sociohistorical context. Moreover, the essay illustrates how this method invites reflexivity, and further, how the reflexive process becomes an active component in data collection and representation.

DISCUSSION QUESTIONS AND ACTIVITIES

1. How does the rise in autobiographical work challenge positivist assumptions about the research process? How does this work extend the qualitative paradigm? How does autoethnography challenge the subject–object, rational–emotional, public–private, and macro–micro dichotomies?

2. What are the issues of validity and trustworthiness that emerge when employing a narrative perspective in the research process? How do these issues differ from traditional conceptions of validity and reliability in positivism and in conventional qualitative research?

3. Try writing an autoethnographic short story about a particular experience where one of your status characteristics played a vital role in your experience (e.g., when gender, race, sexual orientation, religion, age, or health directly influenced some experience). Use this method to try to explore your experience in terms of the setting, the plot, the cultural context, the emotional experience, and your intellectual process, as well as your reflections on the experience. Then reflect on how this method helped illuminate particular aspects of the experience as well as what this method was not able to address or communicate to an external audience.

4. Collect a small sample of data (from ethnographic research or interview work) and experiment with trying to represent it in short-story form, drawing on some of the tenets of fiction. What is your experience of this process, and what issues does it allow you to work through in your own thinking? What does the final product highlight from the data; what might it conceal? Have a peer or colleague read the piece and then discuss his or her understanding of the data, based on the short story.

5. Select an image from a local newspaper. Using the image as a data source, practice an experimental form of writing. What dimensions of the data does this form of writing allow you to access?

SUGGESTED READINGS

Banks, A., & Banks, S. P. (Eds.). (1998). *Fiction and social research: By fire or ice.* New York: AltaMira Press.

This volume was compiled by two researchers who found themselves publishing fiction under pen names and wondering what "truths" were communicated via fiction and nonfiction. Moreover, they wondered why the dualism created between the two prevented so many researchers from producing the kind of writing they truly wanted to create. This collection covers a range of issues and methodological practices that incorporate fiction in the research process.

Bochner, A., & Ellis, C. (Eds.). (2002). *Ethnographically speaking: Autoethnography, literature, and aesthetics.* New York: AltaMira Press.

This comprehensive volume contains articles and essays by some of the most prominent and prolific practitioners of arts-based research. This is an excellent collection of autoethnographic innovations and much more. The chapters are evocatively written, illustrating the issues and practices they detail. A must-read for those interested in arts-based researchers.

Clandinin, D. J. (2007). *Handbook of narrative inquiry: Mapping a methodology.* Thousand Oaks, CA: Sage.

This comprehensive handbook offers a retrospective and prospective review of narrative inquiry. The collection of original works by leading scholars is an excellent reference for researchers across the disciplines working with narrative inquiry.

Ellis, C. (2004). *The ethnographic I: The methodological novel about autoethnography.* New York: AltaMira Press.

This book presents a comprehensive guide to autoethnographic research, addressing both the theoretical and methodological issues as well as providing many rich empirical examples.

Ellis, C., & Bochner, A. (Eds.). (1996). *Composing ethnography: Alternative forms of qualitative writing.* New York: AltaMira Press.

This book provides an excellent resource for those considering alternative methods for writing their qualitative data.

Ely, M., Viz, R., Downing, M., & Anzul, M. (1999). *On writing qualitative research: Living by words.* London: Falmer Press. (Original work published 1997)

This book provides a comprehensive guide to writing qualitative research, including many innovations of storytelling and other creative methods of writing. The book also provides many practical strategies for data analysis, interpretation, and the publication of qualitative research.

SUGGESTED WEBSITES AND JOURNALS

Qualitative Inquiry
  www.sagepub.com/journalsProdDesc.nav?prodId=Journal200797

This journal regularly publishes cutting-edge articles about qualitative methods and methodologies, including many arts-based approaches. *Qualitative Inquiry* routinely provides the most comprehensive collection of innovative qualitative approaches to social research.

Qualitative Report
  www.nova.edu/ssss/QR/index.html

This highly accessible online journal publishes both substantive and methodological articles, including those that cover innovative qualitative methods.

Oral History Review
  ucpressjournals.com/journalSoc.asp?jIssn=0094-0798

The official journal of the Oral History Association, this is an excellent source for articles that rely on the oral history method and related methods such as autoethnography.

CTheory
  www.CTheory.net

This online journal publishes cutting edge research on the borders of popular culture, politics, technology, theory, and methodology. Pieces written in experimental writing formats are often published, making this an excellent source of how to incorporate nontraditional writing, including fiction, into social science research.

Reed Magazine: A Journal of Poetry and Prose
  www.sjsu.edu/reed/open.htm

This is San Jose State University's literary magazine. The journal publishes original poetry and short stories from around the United States.

REFERENCES

Bakhtin, M. M. (1981). *The dialogic imagination: Four essays by M. M. Bakhtin.* Austin: University of Texas Press. (Original work published 1975)

Barone, T., & Eisner, E. (1997). Arts-based educational research. In R. M. Jaeger (Ed.), *Complementary methods for research in education* (2nd ed., pp. 73–116). Washington, DC: American Educational Research Association.

Berger, L. (2001). Inside out: Narrative autoethnography as a path toward rapport. *Qualitative Inquiry, 7*(4), 504–518.

Clandinin, D. J., & Connelly, F. M. (1989). *Narrative and story in practice and research.* (ERIC Document Reproduction Service No. ED309681).

Retrieved from *eric.ed.gov/ERICDocs/data/ericdocs2sql/content_storage_01/00000/9b/80/1f/3d/1f.pdf*

Clandinin, D. J., & Rosiek, J. (2007). Mapping a landscape of narrative inquiry: Borderland spaces and tensions. In D. J. Clandinin (Ed.), *Handbook of narrative inquiry: Mapping a methodology* (pp. 35–75). Thousand Oaks, CA: Sage.

Coffey, A. (1999). *The ethnographic self: Fieldwork and the representation of identity.* London: Sage.

Denzin, N. K. (2001). *Interpretive interactionism: Applied social research methods.* Thousand Oaks, CA: Sage.

Diversi, M. (1998). Glimpses of street life: Representing lived experience through short stories. *Qualitative Inquiry, 4*(2), 131–147.

Dumont, J. (1978). *The headman and I: Ambiguity and ambivalence in the fieldworking experience.* Austin: University of Texas Press.

Ellis, C. (2004). *The Ethnographic I: The methodological novel about autoethnography.* New York: AltaMira Press.

Frank, K. (2000). The management of hunger: Using fiction in writing anthropology. *Qualitative Inquiry, 6*(4), 474–488.

Freeman, M. (2007). Autobiographical understanding and narrative inquiry. In D. J. Clandinin (Ed.), *Handbook of narrative inquiry: Mapping a methodology* (pp. 120–145). Thousand Oaks, CA: Sage.

Gatson, S. N. (2003). On being amorphous: Autoethnography, genealogy, and a multiracial identity. *Qualitative Inquiry, 9*(1), 20–48.

Halpin, T. (1989). Scientific objectivity and the concept of "the other." *Women's Studies International Forum, 12*(3), 285–294.

Harding, S. (1993). Rethinking standpoint epistemology: What is "strong objectivity"? In L. Alcoff & E. Potter (Eds.), *Feminist epistemologies* (pp. 49–82). New York: Routledge.

Harvey, M. R., Mishler, E. G., Koenan, K., & Harney, P. A. (2000). In the aftermath of sexual abuse: Making and remaking meaning in narratives of trauma and recovery. *Narrative Inquiry, 10*(2), 291–311.

Hesse-Biber, S. N., & Leavy, P. (2006a). *Emergent methods in social research.* Thousand Oaks, CA: Sage.

Hesse-Biber, S. N., & Leavy, P. (2006b). *The practice of qualitative research.* Thousand Oaks, CA: Sage.

Jones, K. (2001, May). *Beyond the text: An Artaudian take on the nonverbal clues revealed within the biographical narrative process.* Expanded version of a paper presented at the International Sociological Association International Conference, Kassel, Germany.

Jones, K. (2003). The turn to a narrative knowing of persons: One method explored. *Narrative Studies, 8*(1), 60–71.

Jones, K. (2006). A biographic researcher in pursuit of an aesthetic: The use of arts-based (re)presentations in "performative" dissemination of life stories. *Qualitative Sociology Review, 2*(1). Retrieved from *www.qualitativesociologyreview.org/ENG/index_eng.php*

Kim, J. (2006). For whom the school bell tolls: Conflicting voices inside an alternative high school. *International Journal of Education and the Arts, 7*(6), 1–19.

Labov, W. (2006). Narrative pre-construction. *Narrative Inquiry, 16*(1), 37–45.

Law, J., & Urry, J. (2004). Enacting the social. *Economy and Society, 33*(3), 390–410.

Leavy, P. (2007, August). *Merging feminist principles and art-based methodologies.* Paper presented at the annual conference of the American Sociological Association, New York.

Maines, D. (2001). Writing the self versus writing the other: Comparing autobiographical and life history data. *Symbolic Interaction, 24*(1), 105–111.

McLaurin, S. (2003). Homophobia: An autoethnographic story. *Qualitative Report, 8*(3), 481–486.

Ollerenshaw, J. A., & Creswell, J. W. (2002). Narrative research: A comparison of two restorying data analysis approaches. *Qualitative Inquiry, 8*(3), 329–347.

Pelias, R. J. (2003). The academic tourist: An autoethnography. *Qualitative Inquiry, 9*(3), 369–373.

Pelias, R. J. (2004). *A methodology of the heart: Evoking academic and daily life.* Walnut Creek, CA: AltaMira Press.

Pinnegar, S., & Daynes, J. G. (2007). Locating narrative inquiry historically: Thematics in the turn to narrative. In D. J. Clandinin (Ed.), *Handbook of narrative inquiry: Mapping a methodology* (pp. 3–34). Thousand Oaks, CA: Sage.

Rhodes, C. (2000). Ghostwriting research: Positioning the researcher in the interview text. *Qualitative Inquiry, 6*(4), 511–525.

Rinehart, R. E. (1998). Fictional methods in ethnography: Believability, specks of glass, and Chekhov. *Qualitative Inquiry, 4*(2), 200–224.

Saukko, P. (2000). Between voice and discourse: Quilting interviews on anorexia. *Qualitative Inquiry, 6*(3), 299–317.

Skinner, J. (2003). Montserrat Place and Mons'rat Ncaga: An example of impressionistic autoethnography. *Qualitative Report, 8*(3), 513–529.

Smith, D. (1987). *The everyday world as problematic: A feminist sociology.* Boston: Northeastern University Press.

Tenni, C., Smyth, A., & Boucher, C. (2003). The researcher as autobiographer: Analyzing data written about oneself. *Qualitative Report, 8*(1), 1–12.

Van Maanen, J. (1988). *Tales of the field: On writing ethnography.* Chicago: University of Chicago Press.

Vickers, M. H. (2002). Researcher as storytellers: Writing on the edge—and without a safety net. *Qualitative Inquiry, 8*(5), 608–621.

Wyatt, J. (2005, May). *The telling of a tale: A reading of "A Gentle Going?"* Symposium conducted at the First International Congress of Qualitative Inquiry, Urbana–Champaign, IL.

What Kind of Mother … ?

An Ethnographic Short Story

Karen Scott-Hoy

> How dreadful it will be in those days for pregnant women and nursing mothers!
>
> —MATT. 24:19

A tear trickles down my cheek as I breathe deeply, trying desperately to hold onto this moment; to treasure this time of gentleness, of love, in a day that has been full of horror and pain. As I nurse him, my youngest son's head leans against my chest. His breathing has slowed, and his body becomes heavy in my arms. Fear has left his body for a while. I tuck him into his bed and place his favorite toy alongside him. Automatically, his arm reaches for it and draws it to him, helping him to feel secure and safe. I bend and kiss him gently. We sing our prayer together. At the end he adds, "Please be with the people in America who are sad. … Amen. Goodnight Mum," he drawls sleepily.

Silently, I add my prayer for other would-be terrorists, the people of the Middle East, and for what I fear will occur.

In this story, the author, an Australian mother, questions her reactions to the events of September 11, 2001.

What kind of mother prays for terrorists? "Goodnight sweetheart. Sweet dreams," I reply, although I wonder if that will be possible for anyone tonight, for the world seems a very different, troubled place.

Quietly slipping from the room, I am confronted by a disarming thought. Perhaps the world is not really such a different place; it has just become a less secure place for my family, friends, and me, people in the Western world. Perhaps I am just beginning to understand, to feel, to experience what millions of others in this world live with and through every day. Could it be that the world in which I felt so secure and safe was always an illusion?

I join my older sons in the lounge, where the atmosphere is strained and tense as it has been since the first images of the terrorist attacks on New York and the Pentagon were beamed around the world. Embedded in my mind are the words of the radio announcer on the early morning news and the strain in his voice as he declined to wish early risers the usual "Good morning," for, as he said, "there was nothing 'good' about this morning."

From that moment I had tuned into television reports, in a state of disbelief and shock.

"This is like a movie," says Alex. "It doesn't seem real."

"Yes, it is," I agree.

I realize, like many others here in Australia, most of what my sons know about America and Americans is gleaned through watching movies and television, just as many Americans only know about Australia from watching *Crocodile Dundee*. Maybe that is why, although I see the images and hear the reports, I am finding it so hard to believe, to take in what has happened. In the back of my mind, hope lingers that it is not real, that it has been manufactured or misunderstood like *War of the Worlds*; or maybe I have been conditioned to hope for that Hollywood action hero to somehow rise from the rubble and put everything right.

What kind of mother struggles to tell the difference between fact and fiction, between truth and twaddle?

"Unfortunately, it is real. And it won't have a happy ending," I mumble out loud.

"It's on every channel," Alex says, flicking from station to station.

"I know."

At first I was unsure about letting the children watch the endless reports, but it was on every channel, and so they watched with me. How odd that I should think of stopping them from watching these reports, as many of the action movies they had watched were more violent, more destructive. It must be something to do with the fact that this is real.

"How do you feel when you see that?" I ask as the video of the plane flying into the second tower is screened repeatedly.

"It's weird," Alex replies.

I want to ask what's weird, the notion that someone would fly a plane full of people into a building, or the feeling it gives you watching it, but don't, because "it's weird" seems to sum up how I feel too. I wonder if watching movies has desensitized us to senseless acts of violence and suffering, or if it's just impossible for us to feel anything other than "weird," as the implications of what we are seeing are too overwhelming to deal with right now.

What kind of mother exposes her children to such violence and pain in the name of entertainment?

I've been to "The States," to use the Australian expression, several times, and I've shared the hospitality and friendship of its citizens. My nephew lives in New York. He was my first thought this morning as Australians woke to hear what had happened overnight. He is safe, for now. I have e-mailed other friends to say I am thinking of and praying for them. I don't know what else to do.

I am scheduled to travel to Atlanta next month, and I have been so looking forward to being with friends and attending the National Communication Association convention. As a person and an independent scholar, I value those times immensely, as they enable me to sustain my passion and continue my work. The States are part of my real world, not just my world of entertainment.

As if reading my thoughts, my eldest son looks away from the screen and asks, "Will you still go?"

All day I have been trying to find an answer to that question. I don't want to let terrorism change my life or intimidate me. I want to be defiant. I want to be strong. I want to be close to the people I love, not half a world away. Tears fill my eyes. I want to go.

What kind of mother even contemplates leaving her children at a time like this?

I look at Lachlan and see the fear in his eyes. I say what he wants to hear.

"I don't think so."

He looks relieved and turns back to the screen.

It is now late at night here, early morning in New York. I listen intently as people are interviewed, not because I want to be a voyeur, but because I want to share the burden and understand the pain. Being so far away where life carries on pretty much as usual, I am frightened I might forget for a moment what has happened. I feel somehow that hearing the people's stories will help me make sense of what I see and feel.

A young, fair-haired woman nursing a child is being interviewed. Her dirty face is strained and tear streaked, her eyes seem vacant and withdrawn. Her clothes are covered with dust. The child has in her hand a picture. In large letters is printed the word *MISSING*. I blink hard to clear my blurring vision. The tears roll down my face.

What kind of mother takes her child into a place of such devastation?

I have spent the day calculating the risk of being killed by or involved in a terrorist attack; that mother and child have calculated the chances of survival, of a miracle, of finding hope in the face of hopelessness. I see how she clutches her child. I know how I have struggled here to answer my children's questions; how much harder must it be for her? How do you explain what has happened to a child? Behind her I notice a wall covered with sheets similar to the one her child is holding. There are so many. Having lost a loved one like that, how could you ever say "good-bye" to someone again?

I switch off the television but not the faces, the stories, or the pain.

As the early morning spring sunshine fills the room, I turn the page of the newspaper. "An attack on America is an attack on us." "Australians stand with the U.S. in the War against Terrorism." "Australia pledges troops ... " At 16, my eldest son is too young to be drafted, but I feel afraid. I recall how young Australian men—some just 16—lied about their age to go and fight in 1914. A cold shiver runs down my spine.

What kind of mother sends her sons to war?

On the opposite page, photographs of Osama bin Laden and the hijackers are featured. I wonder how their mothers are feeling, if the mothers' faith is as unshakable as that of their sons. Are they proud of their sons or do they wonder where they went wrong? Dealing with the death of your child seems to me tragic enough, but to know that he was the cause of so many other deaths—I cannot even begin to imagine what that would feel like.

What kind of mother raises sons full of hate and able to kill others?

In this moment, I am reminded of my Eurocentric, Christian worldview. Of course I cannot understand until I am prepared to hear their stories, to listen to what they have to say, to try to suspend my judgments. I see that for some, these acts are perceived to be part of a "holy" war: a war seeking "to make someone pay," to right wrongs. They are acts deeply embedded in and intricately interconnected with the suffering, pain, and power associated with colonialism and oppression, capitalism and poverty, racism and power relations.

Comfortably seated in my kitchen, reading the newspaper and sipping my morning coffee, I realize I hold a position of privilege. Momentarily, I find myself reflecting on this privilege and see that how I live my life may also constitute part of the problem now facing the world; a problem posed—some would say a "wake-up call" delivered—by men prepared to die and kill to make their point.

What kind of mother raises her sons to die for what they believe in?

I have taught my children to stand up for what they think is right. My children have been taught that it's not just what we do, the stategies we employ, that are important, but rather the motivation or meaning we attach to our actions. We talk about what we perceive as injustice in the world and ways we can help make the world a better place. These decisions are commonplace and part of our everyday lives, from simple actions such as recycling rubbish, to making financial commitments to international aid agencies, or our practical hands-on involvement in primary eyecare in the small island nation of Vanuatu in the Southwest Pacific.

Looking back at the photographs of the hijackers, I peer deeply into the eyes of the terrorists trying to see—I don't know what—maybe evidence of evil lurking. I don't see it. They look like anybody looks in their driver's license or I.D. photo. I recall the number of times I have laughed at the "hardened" appearance of friends or relatives in these "mug shots." How can I recognize good and evil? Would I recognize a terrorist if I met one?

I think back to a personal safety campaign—"Stranger Danger"—conducted in our local primary school in response to an increasing number of child molestations and kidnappings. I realize it's been a long time since I offered a ride to a hitchhiker or allowed my child to sit and talk with a stranger without watching them like hawk. My world has changed, not only dramatically as on September 11, but also subtly over a longer period; I just haven't taken the time to notice before. I have allowed "Stranger Danger," fear, and distrust to infiltrate my life and change my behavior.

What kind of mother teaches her children these things?

I turn the page and look down at the photograph of an Afghan mother clutching her child. She is one of many Middle Eastern asylum seekers coming to Australia in boatloads from Indonesia. As I view photographs of Afghanistan and hear stories of unseaworthy boats, of enormous amounts of money paid to corrupt officials and people smugglers, of the horror in their homeland, I wonder if I would have the strength do endure what she has.

What kind of mother smuggles her child out of her homeland?

For some time, these asylum seekers have been viewed by many Australians with suspicion and concern; however, since September 11, they have been perceived as boatloads of potential "sleepers." Images of a sneaky, conniving, manipulative, and coercive people are burned into the minds of an already uneasy public, fueled by media reports of piracy, refusal to leave naval vessels, lack of I.D. papers, hunger strikes and riots, and mothers throwing their children into the sea.

What kind of mother throws her child into the sea?

Some people argue that compassion has given way to fear. Others argue that rational thought must win over irrational desires of "do-gooders," and still others argue that the crisis is not about humanitarian concerns, terrorism, or international goodwill but about shutting down a bad business: the business of people smuggling. "There are legal ways of entering Australia, of applying for asylum, these people are 'queue jumpers,'" says one article. "Desperate people in need of compassion," reads another. "Australia is a multicultural country and richer for it," reports still another.

What kind of mothers do we want in our country?

As I look across at the opposite page of the newspaper, I see that The Wiggles, a popular children's group, are going ahead with their tour to the States. They say it wasn't an easy decision, especially for those with families, but that they must support their fans.

I wonder how you make that choice: fans or families, colleagues or kids? What will these mothers, their wives, tell their children if daddy doesn't come home?

Underneath is a report that the Australian Kangaroos rugby team has canceled its tour because of safety concerns. They are accused of being pathetic wimps.

As I read that, I flinch.

What kind of mother gives into terrorism, cancels her trip, and stays home with her children?

Looking up from the newspaper, I notice Vaughan sitting on the grass in the sun. As I watch, he moves the brightly colored toy cars from place to place, lunging back and forth using the terraced garden, ablaze with spring colors to create different levels. I can hear his chattering and what sounds like singing.

Leaving the newspaper on the table, I make my way outside into the garden.

"That looks like fun!" I exclaim as I approach. "What's happening?"

"The terrorists have just blown up the tourist center and the fire trucks are coming."

I am taken aback at his reply. "Didn't I just hear you singing?"

"No, that was the siren!" he replies.

I smile, but no words will come. I want to scream, to cry out against his loss of innocence. I want singing, not sirens. I want the world to be filled with fairy tales with happy endings. I want good to triumph over evil. I want to be able to meet people and invite them into my home without fear or suspicion. I want to feel safe, to be able to travel to see my friends and colleagues and know that I will come home. I don't want my child playing with terrorists.

Then, as I stop and listen, I realize he is working through and making sense of what has happened in his world through this story, this game. Perhaps if I join in I will find some answers too. I sit beside him. The grass feels cool and still a little damp from the dew. The sun is warm, and the scent of lavender fills the air.

"Can I join you?" I ask.

"Yes. You can be the hospital and look after the sick people," he replies.

"Okay."

He drives over the ambulances.

"What do I do?" I ask.

"Oh. You know … what you always do to make things better."

For a moment I am unsure, caught off guard.

Then I grab him and hold him close to me. We roll over on the grass as I kiss him on the cheek and he shrieks with delight.

"This is what I do to make it better," I laugh.

CHAPTER 3

Poetry and Qualitative Research

> Poetry, I think, is an interruption of silence. The poem makes sense largely
> because it has this space around it. It is inhabiting a part of this space,
> but leaving space around it. So a poem is an interruption of silence, an
> occupation of science; whereas public language is a continuation of noise.
> —BILLY COLLINS, former U.S. Poet Laureate (in Stewart, 2004)

Poems, surrounded by space and weighted by silence, break through the noise to present an essence. Sensory scenes created with skillfully placed words and purposeful pauses, poems push feelings to the forefront capturing heightened moments of social reality as if under a magnifying glass. In contrast to scientific assumptions that science clarifies while art obscures, Pelias (2004) suggests just the opposite:

> Science is the act of looking at a tree and seeing lumber. Poetry is the act of
> looking at a tree and seeing a tree.
>   The alchemy that separates the head from the heart finds no gold.
> (p. 9)

In this regard, the great William Ellery Channing proclaimed:

> Most joyful let the Poet be,
> It is through him that all men see.

Poetry as a research strategy challenges the fact–fiction dichotomy and offers a form for the evocative presentation of data.

The use of poems in the production of social scientific knowledge has increased greatly in recent decades. Somewhere between word and music, poems open a space to represent data in ways that, for some researchers, are attentive to multiple meanings, identity work, and accessing subjugated perspectives. Unlike other forms of expression, in poems the word, sound, and space merge, and this convergence is critical to the construction and articulation of social meaning. Although poetry can be used in various ways during the research process, typically it is employed as a representational form; it is this use of poetry that I explore in this chapter.

Like the practice of qualitative research, poetry is a craft. The poetic representation of social scientific data offers qualitative researchers a representational form that can in some ways be understood as an extension of what they may already do; however, poetry also offers a very particular form in which to interpret and represent human experience and should not be viewed simply as another writing template.

- What is poetic representation?

Poetic Representation

Poetry is a form of representation that relies on the word and lyrical invocation, thus merging two vehicles of expression (Hirshfield, 1997). Poems also usually juxtapose "disparate elements and images together so that each might be considered differently" (Rasberry, 2002, p. 106). In general, poems are highly attentive to space (which includes breath and pauses), using words sparsely in order to paint what I term a *feeling-picture*. Put differently, poems use words, rhythm, and space to create sensory scenes where meaning emerges from the careful construction of both language and silences. In this way, a poem can be understood as evoking a snippet of human experience that is artistically expressed as in a heightened state.

With respect to social research, poems offer an alternative way of presenting data such as those from in-depth interviews or oral history transcripts. Social scientific poems merge the tenets of qualitative research with the craft and rules of traditional poetry. The representation of the data in poetic form is not simply an alternative way of presenting the same information; rather, it can help the researcher evoke different meanings from the data, work through a different set of issues, and help the audience receive the data differently. In this vein, the emergence of poetry within the research process is connected not only to the overall increase in arts-based practices but also to broader epistemological and theoretical insights such as those posed by postmodern and poststructural theory. Feminists and other politically motivated researchers may be interested in the political possibilities of poetry as well as its ability to "stay true" to the speech patterns of interview respondents. As is often the case, the development of new theories and corresponding insights about the social world and the knowledge building process has spawned the development of new research tools (Hesse-Biber & Leavy, 2006, 2008). In addition, there are many genres of poetry that researchers use, each suited to different epistemological views about the research process as well as certain kinds of research questions and objectives. Researchers have also labeled their poetic endeavors with a host of terms.

- Why has poetry emerged as a research tool?
- What are the kinds of poetic forms available to social researchers?

The Emergence of Poetry as a Social Research Method

A recurring theme throughout this book is that methodological innovations typically develop as research paradigms shift, new insights into the social world and practice of research emerge, and theories are developed. In this respect, new methods or approaches to research may come out of a "methods gap" (Hesse-Biber & Leavy, 2006), where methodological innovations are needed in order to address the issues brought forth from new theoretical insights. In the case of poetic representation, this form of expression has emerged in response to shifts toward the qualitative paradigm as well as shifts within that paradigm.

In particular, postmodern theory, postcolonial theory, feminist postmodernism, and feminist poststructuralism have challenged traditional ways of knowing. For example, these schools of thought (generally speaking) are concerned with producing situated and partial knowledge, accessing subjugated voices, decentering authority, and paying attention to the discursive practices that shape experience and our articulation of human experience. As reviewed in Chapter 1, these critical approaches also call attention to the artificiality of binary categories like the rational–emotional split, which historically has dominated knowledge production. These advances in qualitative theorizing directly serve as the context in which poetry has developed as an alternative to traditional prose. As will be discussed in more detail, poetry is a form that itself brings attention to silence (or as a poet might say, to space) and also relies on emotional evocation as a part of meaning-making while simultaneously exposing the fluidity and multiplicity of meaning.

Both Norman Denzin (2003) and Laurel Richardson (1997) have written extensively about the relationship between new theoretical insights, paradigm shifts, and turns toward scientific artistic expression. Richardson has been at the forefront of theorizing about the possibilities of experimental writing and poetic representation, as well as offering methods for the poetic representation of interview data. She uses the term "pleated texts" to conceptualize the multiple layers of meaning that can emerge in between what is there and what is absent. She also distinguishes between *narrative poetry* and *lyric poetry*. In Richardson's framework the former is closer to storytelling, where data gathered from interviews are transformed into a poem that tells the respondent's story, using his or her language. The latter form, lyric poetry, emphasizes moments of emotion and is less concerned with relaying a "story" per se. Richardson explains that this method of writing encourages the researcher to capture the rhythm, tonality, and patterns that comprise speech, in addition to the participants' words themselves. In this way, poetry extends our understanding of "giving voice" to our research collaborators, a key dimension in interpretive and feminist qualitative research.

The idea of narrative poetry, or something similar to it, has also been labeled *research poetry* and *interpretive poetry* (Langer & Furman, 2004), *investigative poetry* (Hartnett, 2003), and *ethnographic poetics* (Brady, 2004; Denzin, 1997). The term "poetic social science" used by Bochner (2000) also speaks to these practices. Ethnographic poetics relies on taking ethnographic data (field notes, memo notes, etc.), meditating on the data (as field researchers typically do), and presenting the results in the form of poems (Denzin, 1997). Similarly, Langer and Furman (2004) discuss interpretive poetry as a method of merging the participant's words with the researcher's perspective. This method of poetic representation therefore offers researchers a new way to account for merging the "voice" of their participants with their own insights, perhaps informed by the larger project of feminism and the like. Because this is consistently a challenge, and one that feminists write about extensively, we can see here how an arts-based practice helps address long-term concerns within the discourse about qualitative practice. Alternatively, Langer and Furman present research poetry as a practice of creating poems from the research participant's words and speech style in order to produce a distilled narrative. Investigative poetry, as described by Hartnett (2003), combines critical ethnography, autobiography, and political underpinnings in service of social justice–oriented goals. Here we can see how new epistemological and theoretical insights regarding the nature of research, the researcher–participant relationship, as well as moves toward research informed by social justice perspectives, have precipitated the investigative method.

A newer and less popular trend in research poetry involves poetry created from literature sources. Researcher-performer Prendergast (2004) terms this practice "literature-voiced research poetry" (p. 75). This method involves using literature as the source from which the researcher creates original poetry. Prendergast grounds this method in the literary tradition of "found poetry" (p. 76). All of her poems in a particular project developed from her work with Herbert Blau's (1990) book *The Audience*. She used the "literature-voiced research poetry" method to "synthesize, process, and make meanings of Blau's theory and how it informs [her] inquiry" (p. 75). The poems, all supported and contextualized with researcher statements, speak to her evolving understanding of audience and performance, central to her career as both a performer and an educator.

- Why might a researcher consider using poetry? What research objectives can poetry help us achieve, and how does this differ from prose?
- How does a researcher put this method into practice?
- What do the interpretive and writing processes entail?

Poetry is an *engaged* method of writing that evokes emotions, promotes human connection and understanding, and may be politically charged (Faulkner, 2005). For these reasons poetry is not for every researcher or every research project; however, when there is an affinity between the research project and the poetic form, this method of representation can capture a unique aspect of the human condition, thereby expanding our understanding of social reality.

As with short stories derived from narrative inquiry, the poetic form is accessible to broader audiences than traditional academic writing opening social scientific knowledge to the public. Former U.S. Poet Laureate Billy Collins notes some of the pleasures of poetry as irony, feeling, drama, imagination, and wordplay (2005, p. xviii). In addition, poetry evokes an emotional response from readers, which may serve particular research objectives.

Sandra Faulkner (2005) suggests that a researcher considers using poetry when prose is insufficient for communicating his or her message. Specifically, she proposes using poetry as a means of provoking "emotional responses in readers and listeners in an effort to produce some shared experience" (p. 9). According to Miles Richardson (1998), poetry is also useful when we want to reveal a moment of truth. This form captures "moments" because "the intensity and compression of poetry emphasizes the vividness" of a moment (Ely, Viz, Downing, & Anzul, 1999, p. 135). Similarly, Laurel Richardson (1997) explains that a part of humanity that may elude the social scientist reveals itself in poetry, allowing the audience to connect with something deep within them (p. 459). The human connection, resonance, and emotionality fostered by poetry results from the unique form poems occupy as compared with other styles of writing. Poems present a porthole onto an experience, one that may be shared by the reader, or one that is new.

For example, bell hooks (1990) examined the poems of Langston Hughes, which, to her, revealed the "erotic longing," lack of fulfillment, and pain that helped shape his life and provide a view into the experience of being a black gay male within that historical and cultural space. hooks's analysis thus suggests that poems can capture intensely subjective "truths" as well as their relation to the larger context. Through their use of language, rhythm, and space, poems represent "the essence of an event" by painting "a scene" that evokes strong imagery and emotions (Ely et al., 1999, p. 135). More than a window onto an aspect of social life, poetry places a *magnifying glass* in front of that reality, where the experience is even bolder than in everyday life. In short, poems can create *a vivid and sensory scene* that *compels the reader,* teaching him or her something about a particular aspect of social experience.

> The poet's business is to create the appearance of "experiences," the semblance of events lived and felt, and to organize them so they constitute a purely and completely experienced reality, a piece of virtual life. (Langer, 1953, p. 212, as quoted in Ely et al., 1999, p. 135)

Although data are condensed in poetic form, this does not minimize its potential to help audiences connect with some aspect of social reality. In fact, the power of a poem as a communicative device is in its ability to dramatically set a sensory scene fostered by attention to the spaces in between words, as well as to those that (literally) appear on the page.

Poems and Identity Research

Researchers engaged in issues pertaining to identity and identity work may find that poetic representation suits their data. In this regard, an excellent example comes from Sandra Faulkner's (2006) work on lesbian –gay–bisexual–transgender–queer (LGBTQ) Jewish Americans' identity negotiation. Faulkner conducted open-ended interviews with 31 people who identify as LGBTQ and Jewish, exploring the question: "What does it mean to be who I am?" This particular group embodies identities that may create conflict or tension, evoke many stereotypes and assumptions, may be at risk for homophobia and anti-Semitism, and each of these identities may be more or less paramount at different times and/or to different people's self concept (Faulkner, 2006). This particular group is also interesting because both identity categories under investigation can be concealed in a way that other identity categories (e.g., race) are less likely to be able to be concealed. Therefore, part of the identity negotiations, or "identity management," of people in this group centers on the extent to which they conceal or reveal their Jewish identity and/or their LGBTQ identity, and how this may differ in different contexts and at different times (Faulkner, 2006). This is clearly a dominant theme in the poems created out of these interviews, as is apparent in the short excerpt that follows.

> Rabbis sigh, throw up their hands: How are gay
> orthodox Jews part of the solution, they're
> part of the problem? Abe says, I'm not *that* Jewish,
> locks himself in a double closet, shut away from religion
> shoves identity into different boxes, passes for parents
> as a devout (but not queer) Jew when in *shul* …

In this study on "identity" the final poems were created directly out of respondents' narratives in a highly collaborative process in which the participants had an opportunity to elaborate or refine the transcripts of their interviews prior to the construction of the final poems. Why was poetic representation used in this project, and how did it suit the researcher's goals?

As discussed earlier, poems reject static or unitary meaning and instead reveal *multiple meanings*. The focus of Faulkner's study is the process of identity negotiation in which LGBTQ Jewish people engage. Accordingly, the poetic representation of data has a tight fit with the research objectives and execution of those objectives. As Faulkner herself explains, "Poetry defies singular definitions and explanations, it mirrors the slipperiness of identity, the difficulty of capturing the shifting nature of who we are and want to be and resonates more fully with the way identity is created, maintained, and altered through our narratives and interactions" (2006, p. 99). Faulkner (2006) goes on to explain that poems allowed her simultaneously to expose how identities are traditionally represented and to expand the presentation of complex identities in relevant academic literatures. In addition, the poems provoke emotional engagement and human connection between the author, the person being represented, and the audience—a key facet of identity research with a social action intention. This kind of engagement and connection challenges readers to transgress stereotypical ways of thinking about different groups and is therefore compatible with social justice motivations. The "truths" that come forth in poems may also be an important part of how this research helps us understand how identity management happens with respect to "concealable identities" (Crocker, Major, & Steele, 1998) and how disclosure, partial disclosure, or nondisclosure of those identities may be linked to fears about homophobia and anti-Semitism, which are themselves more or less pronounced in different contexts and at different times.

Poetry can also help us understand other aspects of identity and experience that may be linked to a range of particular circumstances or experiences, including health issues. For example, Zenobia C. Y. Chan employs poetry as a means of understanding the complex issues surrounding eating disorders in females. Drawing on her standpoint as a woman with cross-disciplinary training in nursing, social work, women's studies, and qualitative research, Chan found herself frustrated with the limited focus of much of the literature on eating disorders. To address this perceived gap, Chan (2003) used poetry as a means of opening the subject up from a literary perspective. Her poem, simply titled "Anorexia," touches on many issues ranging from the social context in which eating disorders emerge, to the personal pain of parents coping with their daughters' eating disorders, to the behavioral aspects of eating disorders (e.g., food restriction, food obsession), as well as issues pertaining to the anorexic identity (potentially far more complex than the literature to date has suggested). The author follows a format of four-line stanzas; each line of the stanza begins with a particular letter of the alphabet and the lines of the first and last stanzas begin with the letter "A" (the poem begins with the word "anorexia" and the last line of the last stanza begins with the word "affliction"). A brief excerpt from the poem follows:

> Enduring her fasting is destroying her parents,
> Ending her anorexia is one day foreseeable.
> Eating is her enemy.
> Eccentricities in eating habits are her representation.

This poem, carefully crafted in both form and content, is able to bring forth a wide range of issues pertaining to our understanding of eating disorders including sociocultural issues, psychological issues, family issues, health issues, and identity negotiation. Furthermore, the poem is able to touch on all of these issues in a condensed way that highlights each of them while showing their interconnectivity. Moreover, the poem is evocative and seems to represent many individuals with this affliction while remaining deeply personal and subjective as if it represents one woman's narrative. In this way, poems are able to tap into the collective and personal, or the macro and micro, making them sociologically engaged and also compelling for the reader. Cynthia Cannon Poindexter's (2002) work, reprinted later in this chapter, explores similar issues pertaining to health, identity, and culture in her research that uses poetry as a means of communicating how one couple experiences an HIV diagnosis.

Poems and Autoethnography

Poetry is therefore one of the forms that autoethnographies can take, as there is a congruence between the evocative capabilities of poetry and autoethnography. In this vein, Ronald J. Ricci (2003) used poetry to present autoethnographic data that revealed his childhood memories of growing up with two distinct family cultures. He combined autoethnography and poetry in order to provide meaning, evoke emotion, and engage in reflexive practice.

I have recently begun using poetry as an interpretive strategy and representational form in my own autoethnographic work. As noted elsewhere in this book, I have been conducting in-depth interview research on the subject of body image and sexual identity. As is often the case with qualitative research, I have garnered data on a range of unanticipated dimensions of my topic.

For example, I have been struck by how the women interviewed think about their ideal romantic relationships in the context of fantasy-based media images of women, sexuality, and love. Moreover, I have noted many of the disjunctures between their fantasies and their "real-life" relationships, particularly as they experienced loss and/or betrayal. During my traditional qualitative data analysis and interpretation, which consisted of memo note-taking, computer-assisted analysis, and theoretical note-taking, I was drawn to include my own experiences with the data collected on these "unanticipated" dimensions. To do so I began creating poems informed by the interview data, autobiographical data, and media sources (such as "entertainment news" and children's popular media). Three of the resulting poems follow:

Barbie Bandits and Beauty Queens

I am on a witch hunt.
    Where, where have all the girls gone?
Barbie Bandits and Beauty Queens
we were sold a line, a cosmetic line history
    Where have the girls' stories disappeared to?

Spells and Potions
Rolling Pins and Pies

write her out, white her out, her story is hiding out

The Patriarchy runs this show spectacular
Their media-makers spin world-wide webs
a Bethlehem tale of two genders
flawlessly furnished,
    with Barbie Bandits and Beauty Queens

The Feminine Betrayal of Love and Fame

I was watching TV when he told me. *Entertainment Tonight,* I think.
    A special edition.
Mickey Mouse Club Trainwrecks.
Toxic.
Feminine betrayal.

Such a fool I thought
How I spun round and round shaped by his hands
He left me to reel
Nowhere to found at the Lost and Found

How I would sway
For this man, this man spinning a dream sure to betray
For him the thrill could only be taken
Awaken
from the nightmare of his lies I dare

the residual is the price to pay
for what we long to give away
our starlet seduces as she screws
the lens that exploits its own muse

I still spin, now in despair
searching for but an unfinished self's trace
she is desperate for Hollywood's glare
I hear the new girl is in our place
    we spin
    we spin in this vacuous space

Fairytale Undone

fairytale lies
slipping through the cracks
between which he carefully placed   stolen facts

        Cinderella lost her slipper
        as she tripped running away
        shattering the glass
        tripping me on my way

a fantasy that was built
in a house built on lies
and what lies beneath, in the lies beneath
begin to creep through
squeezing between the cracks
a lost battleground of surrendered facts
push through my feet
I start to retreat
into me one lone splinter
the white noise of our winter

Poems and Collective Biography Research

Poems may also be used in collective memory and collective biography work, whether the data are in the form of multiple individual interviews or coauthored narratives, or rather the result of focus-group interviews and the like. Here I turn to an excellent example from Susanne Gannon's (2001) research in which she became "paralyzed" (metaphorically speaking) when faced with the task of analyzing the stories from a women's group, which they referred to as "memory texts," that had developed over the course of many workshops in which Gannon participated. Her dilemma was that she was charged with presenting a "collective" analysis, yet as she began traditional qualitative methods of analysis and interpretation she soon realized that she was "sliding" into individual stories tacked on to each other. To contend with this challenge Gannon changed her method of analysis; drawing on the work of Laurel Richardson she began to craft poems.

Using the "memory texts" that developed in the workshops, Gannon constructed two poems about the "life/lives of a collective girl" (p. 791). The analysis process consisted of drawing out central images, words, and ideas from the whole and then preserving each woman's "voice" (via syntax, rhythm, and language), which were then interwoven to create a collective or composite woman while maintaining the individual threads that comprise her. Gannon's reflexive and candid discussion of this process illustrates the effectiveness of this arts-based approach, as well as the value of being open to recognizing when something isn't working and then adapting accordingly. Researchers who delve into arts-based methods often have to let go of preconceived notions and design plans and remain flexible and open to revision. Contrary to common critiques, Skinner, Leggo, Irvin, Gouzouasis, and Grauer (2006) suggest that flexibility is a core strength of arts-based approaches.

Poems and Subjugated Perspectives, Oppression, and Unearned Privileges

The final reason why a researcher might use poetry brings us back to the issue of accessing subjugated knowledge and the experience of those who are disenfranchised. Here the specific form that poetry occupies becomes paramount to the articulation of marginalized voices. I am referring to "spaces" in poetry, which are integral to their form. In poems meaning is imparted in the space as well as the words. Space and breath are inextricably bound to meaning production. In this way, the spaces that partly comprise poems are *weighted*. Mazzei (2003) offers the idea of "a poetic understanding of silence," which purposefully conceptualizes silences as "inhabited" (p. 356). Mazzei refers to Rich and Lehman's (1996) commentary about white poets who write about race. They assert, "Relationships of race and power exist in their poems most often as a silence or a muffled subtext" (p. 32). The poetic form can therefore help us access those aspects of a hierarchical society that may be further rendered invisible in traditional forms of scientific writing. In other words, poetry can help us access the *subtext* that helps shape our experience, perception, and understanding of social reality; this is particularly salient in a society in which many are forced to the peripheries of the dominant order and within which others enjoy the "unearned privileges" associated with their dominant status, privileges that the recipient is exonerated from recognizing.

- How do researchers create poems out of their data?
- What do the interpretive and writing processes entail?

Analysis, Interpretation, and Writing Research Poems

As with any other form of qualitative research, there are many strategies for the interpretation and writing up of data. Procedures should meet particular research objectives as well as the epistemological and theoretical commitments underscoring the project. In the Rasberry example on "collective biography," in which individual narratives became the threads woven as one collective woman's story, we already gleaned a sense of one methodological approach to analysis. With this said, I now review one broad technique social scientists often employ (on a continuum) as they make sense of and represent their data: poetic transcription.

Poetic Transcription and Grounded Theory

Poetic transcription is an approach to analysis and writing derived from a grounded theory perspective (although not precisely the same), where code categories develop inductively out of the data. In the case of interview data, for example, a researcher interested in poetic transcription first studies the interview transcripts looking for themes and recurring language, then draws exact words and phrases out of the data. The selected words and phrases become the basis of the poem. In addition to using respondents' language, this approach also preserves narrators' speech patterns (Faulkner, 2005; Glesne, 1997). This technique ultimately relies on extensive thematic coding, constituting a process of reduction where single words may come to represent segments of an interview transcript. Although participants' language serves as the frame for the poem, the researcher may also incorporate his or her own language; for example, part of their dialogue during the interview may be infused into the poem. Glesne (1997) classifies poetic transcription as presenting a "third voice" that comes from the conversation between the respondent and researcher and develops during interpretation. Likewise, insights from a literature review or theoretical scholarship may be a part of this third voice. Again, we can see how poetry offers qualitative practitioners a way to address the tension between commitments to participants' voice as well as their own insights and political motivations—a tension frequently categorized under the terms *authorship* and *authority* in existing literature.

According to Madison (2005), this approach developed out of feminist and multiculturalist concerns with respect to allowing the narrator's voice to emerge, concerns that are central to the larger project of feminism. Researchers committed to accessing subjugated voices might be especially inclined toward this interpretation style. Furthermore, as many critical scholars believe, the respondent's narrative occurs at the point of articulation and therefore capturing the speech style of the narrator not only preserves his or her voice but also assists in communicating the performative aspects of the interview (Calafell, 2004; Faulkner, 2005). Whether or not poetic transcription is used, variations of grounded theory analysis may prove useful as a researcher tries to interpret his or her data and represent them in a manner that retains the speaker's voice, or *the sound* of the interview conversation itself. Moreover, a grounded-theory approach to interpretation adds a built-in dimension of authenticity to the data per the mandates of traditional qualitative research.

The following empirical example illustrates one approach to analysis and representation. The data come from a study about the relationship between sexual identity and body image among college-age females and males (this research was supported by a grant from the Foundation for the Society for the Scientific Study of Sexuality). For this example I focus on the 18 female participants who self-identified as bisexual, heterosexual, or homosexual. Each participated in an in-depth, open-ended interview. While each participant was asked similar questions aimed at probing a defined set of issues, the interviewees had ample freedom to discuss issues of import to them and participate in shaping the flow of conversation. The interviews were then transcribed verbatim, and the interviewees were all assigned a number (and the transcripts cleaned of identifying personal information) and then systematically coded by two coders for intercoder reliability. The result was a lengthy list of metacodes (large code categories) including codes such as Attractiveness, Body Image, Family, Dating, and so forth. Under each metacode category there was a larger list of smaller, more specific code categories such as Attractiveness Ideals Others, Attractiveness Ideals Self, Body Satisfaction, Body Dissatisfaction, First Date, Date Preparation, and so on.

Below is a copy of the coded transcripts that address the smaller code category of "Breasts," which fell under the metacode category of "Body Image." Five out of 18 respondents chose to discuss this topic, which they were not specifically asked about, and therefore this small section of the coded data is useful for this kind of illustration.

13

AND MY BOOBS!!! I WISH MY BOOBS WERE BIGGER!

(Interviewer) OK, why?

I don't know. [*giggle*] 'cause ... I don't know. I, I don't know, maybe it's the images I see ... I guess. It's probably what it is, you know? Seeing women my size, 5 foot 2, skinny with like bigger breasts, for no reason. You know? They're skinny you know, but they have like bigger boobs! I don't know, I guess I wish I had a little cleav ... (cleavage) to fill out some of my shirts. [*giggle*] I guess that's all. ...

8

Yeah, I heart lingerie. I never used to and I have small breasts, and I never used to wear bras with underwire or push-up bras or anything like that. I just used to wear like, you know, strips of fabric that would cover the nipples. [*Laughing.*] But like, when did I start wearing real bras? I think junior year of college. No? Sophomore year of college, I actually started wearing real bras. And like that's pretty late I think for a girl, uh, and I did it because, well, when I wasn't wearing bras it was because like I wanted my body to look the way that it is and I wanted to just present my body in the form that it was and I didn't want to pretend to ever, like, other people. But I felt like a lot of girls who did that were like, it reflected on their appearance, but like the past few years I fell in love with lingerie and like how it can accentuate the good parts. And I realized that it doesn't reflect on character and your character is there regardless of how you shape your body. It can exist, independently anyway, so you know, I heart lingerie. But I heart my small boobs, like I like them the way they are.

17

(Interviewer) What do you think are the good parts of our body?

Um, well ... Um, I think that, I have nice [*laugh*] breasts [*laughs*] so I definitely wear tight shirts so they look good. Um, yeah!

I feel that society pushes us to be like, tall, and skinny with huge boobs and have the perfect body and look like Jessica Simpson and look like all of the ads with the models with perfect bodies in them.

You watched MTV all the time, even the people on *Real World* are gorgeous, like they all have boob jobs and are so skinny and the guys are bricks, and so I think that when I realized I had a problem, everyone doesn't look like that.

14

I hate my boobs!

(Interviewer) Why do you hate your boobs?

Because they are too saggy and too far apart! [*Giggle*] and I want to get a boob job, when I get ... 'cause I want to be a lawyer, and so like when I get my first big case I'm gonna buy fake boobs.

3

I would really enjoy it if I had bigger boobs, I think if I completely filled out a B I would be happy with that but instead I am on the smaller side of the B which is small.

(Interviewer) So you would like bigger boobs?

Yeah, or at least like I don't know I just don't feel like I have the ideal boobs.

(Interviewer) What are the ideal boobs?

Well, I think shapely, and they have a certain nipple size that is perfect, I don't know [*laughs*].

(Interviewer) Where did you get this idea from?

Umm, well, I got to say, probably man's portrayal of what they like, 'cause I'd say women if they had to say what they like, they'd like smaller boobs, because bigger boobs cause problems, you know, when you exercise they are all jiggly or what not. So I would have to say it's definitely a male want.

As you can see, all of the typical procedures for gathering and analyzing qualitative interview data have been followed up until this point. Let's look at how these kind of data can be further analyzed and represented in poetic form. At this point I go back to the transcript and highlight with **bold type** some of the words that capture the essence of what these women are conveying. I use data from each of the respondents. The highlighted transcript follows.

13

AND MY BOOBS!!! I WISH MY BOOBS WERE BIGGER!

(Interviewer) OK, why?

I don't know. [*giggle*] 'cause ... I don't know. I, I don't know, maybe it's the images I see ... I guess. It's probably what it is, you know? Seeing women my size, 5 foot 2, skinny with like **bigger breasts**, for no reason. You know? They're skinny you know, but they have like **bigger boobs!** I don't know, I guess I wish I had **a little cleav** ... (cleavage) to fill out some of my shirts [*giggle*] I guess that's all ...

8

Yeah, **I heart lingerie. I never used to** and **I have small breasts,** and I never used to wear bras with underwire or push-up bras or anything like that. I just used to wear like, you know, strips of fabric that would cover the nipples. [*Laughing.*] But like, when did I start wearing real bras? I think junior year of college. No? Sophomore year of college, I actually started wearing real bras. And like that's pretty late I think for a girl, uh, and I did it because, well, when I wasn't wearing bras it was because like I wanted my body to look the way that it is and I wanted to just present my body in the form that it was and I didn't want to pretend to ever, like, other people. But I felt like a lot of girls who did that were like, it reflected on their appearance, but like the past few years I fell in love with lingerie and like how it can accentuate the good parts. And I realized that it doesn't reflect on character and your character is there regardless of how you shape your body. It can exist, independently anyway, **so you know, I heart lingerie. But I heart my small boobs, like I like them the way they are.**

17

(Interviewer) What do you think are the good parts of our body?

Um, well ... Um, I think that, I have nice [*laugh*] **breasts** [*laughs*] so I definitely wear tight shirts so they look good. Um, yeah!

I feel that **society pushes us to be like, tall, and skinny with huge boobs** and have the perfect body and look like Jessica Simpson and look like all of the ads with the models with perfect bodies in them.

You watched MTV all the time, even the people on *Real World* are gorgeous, like they all have **boob jobs** and are **so skinny** and the **guys are bricks,** and so I think that when I realized I had a problem, everyone doesn't look like that.

14

I hate my boobs!

(Interviewer) Why do you hate your boobs?

Because they are **too saggy** and **too far apart!** [*Giggle*] and **I want to get a boob job,** when I get ... 'cause I want to be a lawyer, and so like when I get my first big case I'm **gonna buy fake boobs.**

3

I would really enjoy it **if I had bigger boobs,** I think if I completely filled out a B I would be happy with that but instead I am on the smaller side of the B which is small.

(Interviewer) So you would like bigger boobs?

Yeah, or at least like I don't know **I just don't feel like I have the ideal boobs.**

(Interviewer) What are the ideal boobs?

Well, I think **shapely,** and they have **a certain nipple size that is perfect,** I don't know [*laughs*].

(Interviewer) Where did you get this idea from?

Umm, well, I got to say, **probably man's portrayal of what they like,** 'cause I'd say women if they had to say what they like, they'd like smaller boobs, because **bigger boobs cause problems,** you know, when you exercise they are **all jiggly** or what not. So I would have to say it's definitely **a male want.**

The resulting poem follows:

... And My Boobs
bigger breasts
bigger boobs
too saggy
too far apart
all jiggly

tall and skinny with huge boobs
society pushes us
man's portrayal
a male want
    guys are bricks

I have small breasts
but I heart my small boobs

I like them the way they are

I want to get a boob job
gonna buy fake boobs

If I had bigger boobs
bigger boobs
    a certain nipple size that is perfect

I just don't feel like   I have the ideal boobs

In this example, only the respondents' exact language was used in the final representation; however, the researcher selected the parts of the data that would be used and therefore retained interpretive control. The poem dramatically reduces the data and simultaneously emphasizes aspects of it that, when crafted, become quite emotional and represent very personal experiences that are also weaved together to represent a composite woman. Furthermore, although brief, the poem addresses the macro context in which women have these experiences and develop these self-concepts, particularly patriarchy, media, and the cosmetic surgery industry, and is thus a way of linking micro and macro levels of analysis.

Now that analysis and interpretation are clearer, it is important to consider issues of authenticity and validity.

- How can social scientific poems be evaluated? What criteria can be used to help judge the validity of research poems? How do these validity measures bump up against more traditional approaches?

Issues of Trustworthiness and Validity in Social Scientific Poems

As with all of the arts-based practices reviewed in this volume, a primary concern regarding the poetic representation of social scientific data revolves around the criteria by which the research community and public might judge such work. More specifically, traditional measures of validity, even those within the qualitative paradigm, may not be effective in evaluating research poems. Although validity and related issues emerge in discussions about all arts-based practices, the use of poetry is a particularly new innovation and thus the subject of premature dismissal by some and intense scrutiny by others. What is important to understand when contemplating important issues of validity and authenticity is that this kind of data cannot be judged by positivist standards, and at times cannot even be evaluated by traditional qualitative "interpretive" standards (in their conventional configuring). However, as discussed in Chapter 1, the emergence of new methods, guided by theoretical innovations, creates a space for us to reconsider matters of evaluation with regard to the specifics of the new approaches. Working through these complex issues therefore strengthens our understanding of concepts like validity and promotes advancement within the qualitative paradigm.

Although still a relatively new area, there are some basic guidelines for attaining trustworthiness in research poems. First, poetry is a complex artistic craft with its own set of normative practices and literary rules. It is therefore a mistake for researchers to assume they can write poems, or do so easily, simply because they want to "experiment" with the form without paying attention to craft in its own right. Rather, researchers embarking on a poetic project need to study the tradition of poetry, learn the rules of poetry (Percer, 2002), and begin to understand the hard work that goes into *crafting* poems. In short, the use of poetry in research increases rigor in the interpretation and writing processes, it does not diminish it. Moreover, attention to the poetic form itself enhances the aesthetic qualities of the work, which in turn increases positive audience response; the audience response is itself a validity checkpoint in arts-based research.

Beyond studying poetry as a craft so that one learns "the rules" as well as those of social research, poems can be judged based on their ability to evoke emotions, produce connections, create a scene that *feels* truthful, and inspire political or socially conscious action (Faulkner, 2005a). Drawing on the work of Richardson (2000) and Bochner (2000), Faulkner suggests that we pay special attention to the emotional undertones of the poem and the feelings they produce for the audience. For Richardson the emotional response of readers is critical, while Bochner asks the reader to contemplate the truthfulness of the emotions expressed by the poet-researcher. In other words, when reading a research poem, what does your internal monitor say? What is your emotional, gut-level response? How does the poem promote issues of social justice or understanding across difference? Does the poem call forth something from your experience or help shed light on an experience that is unfamiliar to you? These are the kinds of questions we can ask ourselves as we evaluate particular poems.

The role the researcher's "internal monitor" plays in his or her research is central within ontological and epistemological debates about knowledge-building. As reviewed in Chapter 1, feminists have been at the forefront of challenging the dichotomous thinking that guides positivism. In particular, feminists have challenged the rational–emotional dualism (Sprague & Zimmerman, 1993) while also illustrating how emotions infuse all aspects of research, often serving as the impetus for a research project (Jaggar, 1989). Situated in this context, the call to emotions as a validity checkpoint or source by which to consider authenticity can be viewed as an extension of the work of many qualitative feminists. I therefore identify the privileging of emotions as another point of convergence between the project of feminism and the scientific adaptation of poetry.

Another criterion by which we might evaluate poems comes from the field of poetry itself, a field partly shaped by debates over how "accessible" poems should be with respect to clarity of meaning. Billy Collins suggests that the idea of "accessibility" can be reconceptualized as "easy to enter" (2005, p. xiv). In this regard, Collins suggests that poems should be "easy to enter" so that readers have an entrée into the meanings contained within them.

> An accessible poem has a clear entrance, a front door through which the reader may pass into the body of the poem or whose overall "accessibility"— i.e.: availability of meaning—remains to be seen and may vary widely. (2005, p. xiv)

This principle can be applied to social scientific poems as well.

Beyond the measures already reviewed, Sandra Faulkner (2005a) provides the following list of scientific and artistic criteria, followed by her assessment of "poetic criteria."

Scientific Criteria	*Artistic Criteria*
depth	compression of data
authenticity	understanding of craft
trustworthiness	social justice
understanding of human	moral truth
experience	emotional verisimilitude
reflexivity	evocation
usefulness	sublime
articulation of craft/method	empathy
ethics	

Poetic Criteria
artistic concentration
embodied experience
discovery/surprise
conditional
narrative truth
transformation

As you can see, the measures of trustworthiness used to evaluate qualitative research and those used to judge the quality of artistic poetry merge in Faulkner's final list. In this way, "poetic criteria" do not privilege social scientific or artistic ways of creating and knowing "truth(s)"; rather, proposing the hybridization or merging of the two creates a *third space* for contemplating what counts as knowledge, paralleling the "third voice" produced by poetic transcription. In this way, working through the challenges of creating criteria by which to judge and compare research poems is also a way for social scientists to challenge and expand standard definitions of knowledge itself. Accordingly, poetry is both a style of representation as well as a vehicle through which the academic/research community can engage in larger questions about the nature of social research, truth, and knowledge.

Checklist of Considerations

When considering using poetry for the representation of your data it may help to ask yourself the following:

✓ What are the goals of my study, and how will poetic analysis and representation foster those goals? How will the poetic form help get at and reveal issues in ways that differ from traditional prose?

✓ What do I want the poems to evoke in readers?

✓ What views regarding the nature of knowledge are underpinning my research, and are these views consistent with the use of poetry?

✓ How will I construct poems out of my data? What is my plan for analysis, interpretation, and writing? For example, to what extent, if any, will a grounded-theory approach be used? How will existing scholarship inform the writing process?

✓ How will I think about issues pertaining to validity? How does my analysis procedure build authenticity and trustworthiness?

Conclusion

Consider the issues that arose in this chapter with respect to the nature of knowledge-building, experience, and emotionality in social science as you read the article that follows this chapter. Cynthia Cannon Poindexter's piece about how a couple copes with an HIV diagnosis shows the strengths of poetry as a research method. Moreover, her research indicates that significant and highly sensitive subject matter can be addressed with arts-based practices.

DISCUSSION QUESTIONS AND ACTIVITIES

1. Why might a researcher studying sexual harassment in the workplace, the experience of racial or sexual prejudice, or homophobia as experienced in a gay or lesbian family consider using poetry as a research tool? How are these kinds of issues addressed by poetry? What can poems help us access with respect to these topics that traditional qualitative methods of representation often distort or obscure?

2. How might poetry assist a researcher who is interested in studying the identity management practices in the high school, family, and peer contexts of first-generation Americans who live with a parent or parents born in a different country?

3. Use the data provided in Appendix 3.1 and perform a poetic analysis, ultimately representing the data as a poem. (These data are a part of the same coded interviews on body images and sexual identity used earlier. These data come from the code category Attractiveness Ideals Self).

SUGGESTED READINGS

Ely, M., Viz, R., Downing, M., & Anzul, M. (1999). *On writing qualitative research: Living by words.* London: Falmer Press. (Original work published 1997)

This book provides a comprehensive guide to writing qualitative research, including many innovations of poetry and other creative methods of writing. The book also provides many practical strategies for data analysis, interpretation, and the publication of qualitative research.

Leedy, J. J. (Ed.). (1985). *Poetry as healer: Mending the troubled mind.* New York: Vanguard Press.

This classic anthology is filled with essays covering a range of topics pertinent to the poetry–healing relationship.

National Association for Poetry Therapy. (2006). *The National Federation for Bibio/ Poetry Therapy Guide to Training Requirements.* Delray Beach, FL: Author.

This is a comprehensive guide for those contemplating entering the field of poetry therapy.

vanMeenen, K., Rossiter, C., & Adams, K. (Eds.). (2001). *Giving sorrow word: Poems of strength and solace.* Delray Beach, FL: National Association for Poetry Therapy.

This collection includes the poetry of internationally known poets as well as a guide for individuals and professionals, reviewing how reading, writing, and discussing poetry can be healing and foster individual growth. The collection also features brief commentaries and writing activities linked to each specific poem.

SUGGESTED WEBSITES AND JOURNALS

Alba: A Journal of Short Poetry
   www.ravennapress.com/alba/submit.html

This journal, published biannually, accepts original poetry submissions (only via e-mail and only in the body of e-mails). Interested poets can submit short poems (not more than 12 lines) to *albaeditor@yahoo.com.* The journal prefers free verse as opposed to established forms, although all styles are considered.

Reed Magazine: A Journal of Poetry and Prose
   www.sjsu.edu/reed/open.htm

This is San Jose State University's literary magazine. The journal publishes original poetry and short stories from around the United States.

Journal of Poetry Therapy: The Interdisciplinary Journal of Practice, Theory, Research, and Education (JPT)

JPT is a peer-reviewed interdisciplinary journal sponsored by the National Association for Poetry Therapy. The journal publishes full-length articles about the use of the language arts in therapeutic practices. Articles can be primarily theoretical, historical, literary, clinical, or evaluative. Poems and short reports (four to seven pages) are also published.

National Association for Poetry Therapy
   poetrytherapy.org

The website for this association contains many features of interest, including membership information, books, conferences, events, and many other resources. Of particular interest is *The Museletter,* the official newsletter of this organization, which is published three times a year. The newsletter spans many topics, including book reviews, information about arts-based therapies, and articles about poetry therapy.

REFERENCES

Blau, H. (1990). *The audience*. Baltimore: Johns Hopkins University Press.

Bochner, A. (2000). Criteria against ourselves. *Qualitative Inquiry, 6,* 278–291.

Brady, I. (2004). In defense of the sensual: Meaning construction in ethnography and poetics. *Qualitative Inquiry, 10,* 622–644.

Calafell, B. M. (2004). Disrupting the dichotomy: 'Yo Soy Chicana/o?' in the new Latina/o south. *Communication Review, 7,* 175–204.

Chan, Z. C. Y. (2003). A poem: Anorexia. *Qualitative Inquiry, 9*(6), 956–957.

Collins, B. (2005). *180 more: Extraordinary poems for every day.* New York: Random House.

Crocker, J., Major, B., & Steele, C. (1998). Social stigma. In D. Gilbert, S. Fiske, & G. Lindzey (Eds.), *Handbook of social psychology* (pp. 504–553). Boston: McGraw-Hill.

Denzin, N. K. (1997). *Interpretive ethnography: Ethnographic practices for the 21st century.* Thousand Oaks, CA: Sage.

Denzin, N. K. (2003). *Performance ethnography: Critical pedagogy and the politics of culture.* Thousand Oaks, CA: Sage.

Ely, M., Viz, R., Downing, M., & Anzul, M. (1999). *On writing qualitative research: Living by words.* London: Falmer Press.

Faulkner, S. L. (2005, May). *How do you know a good poem?: Poetic representation and the case for criteria.* Symposium conducted at the First International Conference of Qualitative Inquiry, Urbana–Champaign, Illinois.

Faulkner, S. L. (2006). Reconstruction: LGBTQ and Jewish. *International and Intercultural Communication Annual, 29,* 95–120.

Gannon, S. (2001). Representing the collective girl: A poetic approach to a methodological dilemma. *Qualitative Inquiry, 7*(6), 787–800.

Glesne, C. (1997). That rare feeling. Re-presenting research through poetic transcription. *Qualitative Inquiry, 3,* 202–222.

Hartnett, S. J. (2003). *Incarceration nation: Investigative prison poems of hope and terror.* Walnut Creek, CA: AltaMira Press.

Hesse-Biber, S. N., & Leavy, P. (2006). *Emergent methods in social research.* Thousand Oaks, CA: Sage.

Hesse-Biber, S. N., & Leavy, P. (2008). Pushing on the methodological boundaries: The growing need for emergent methods within and across the disciplines. In S. N. Hesse-Biber & P. Leavy (Eds.), *Handbook of emergent methods.* New York: Guilford Press.

Hirshfield, J. (1997). *Nine gates: Entering the mind of poetry.* New York: HarperCollins.

hooks, b. (1990). *Yearning: Race, culture, and politics.* Boston: South End Press.

Jaggar, A. (1989). Love and knowledge: Emotion in feminist epistemology. *Qualitative Inquiry, 32,* 151–172.

Langer, S. (1953). *Feeling and form.* New York: Scribner.

Langer, C. L., & Furman, R. (2004, March). Exploring identity and assimilation: Research and interpretive poems [19 paragraphs]. *Forum Qualitative Sozialforschung/Forum: Qualitative Social Research* [Online journal], *5*(2). Available at *www.qialitativeresearch.net/fqs-texte/2-04/2-04langerfurman-e.htm*

Madison, D. S. (2005). *Critical ethnography: Method, ethics, and performance.* Thousand Oaks, CA: Sage.

Mazzei, L. A. (2003). Inhabited silences: In pursuit of a muffled subtext. *Qualitative Inquiry, 9*(3), 355–368.

Pelias, R. J. (2004). *A methodology of the heart: Evoking academic and daily life.* Walnut Creek, CA: AltaMira Press.

Percer, L. H. (2002, June). Going beyond the demonstrable range in educational scholarship: Exploring the intersections of poetry and research. *Qualitative Report, 7*(2). Retrieved from *www.nova.edu/ssss/QR/QR7-2/hayespercer.html*

Poindexter, C. C. (2002). Research as poetry: A couple experiences HIV. *Qualitative Inquiry, 8,* 707–714.

Prendergast, M. (2004). "Shaped like a question mark": Found poetry from Herbert Blau's *The Audience. Research in Drama Education, 9*(1), 73–92.

Rasberry, G. W. (2002). Imagine, inventing a data-dancer. In C. Bagley & M. B. Cancienne (Eds.), *Dancing the data* (pp. 106–120). New York: Peter Lang.

Ricci, R. J. (2003). Autoethnographic verse: Nicky's boy: A life in two worlds. *Qualitative Report, 8*(4), 591–596.

Rich, A., & Lehman, D. (1996). *The best American poetry.* New York: Scribner Paperback Poetry.

Richardson, L. (1997). Skirting a pleated text: De-disciplining an academic life. *Qualitative Inquiry, 3,* 295–304.

Richardson, L. (2000). Evaluating ethnography. *Qualitative Inquiry, 6,* 253–255.

Richardson, M. (1998). Poetics in the field and on the page. *Qualitative Inquiry, 4,* 451–462.

Skinner, A., Leggo, C., Irwin, R., Gouzouasis, P., & Grauer, K. (2006). Arts-based education research dissertations: Reviewing the practices of new scholars. *Canadian Journal of Education, 29*(4), 1223–1270.

Sprague, J., & Zimmerman, M. (1993). Overcoming dualisms: A feminist agenda for sociological method. In P. England (Ed.), *Theory on gender/feminism on theory* (pp. 255–279). New York: DeGruyter.

Stewart, R. (2004). The end of boredom: An interview with Billy Collins. *New Letters: A Magazine of Writing and Art, 70*(2), 143–159.

APPENDIX 3.1

5

Okay. So what you said before, the shallow reason is that you do some of these things to be attractive to others, what is like, what would make you attractive? What is your goal, what would you want to be to be attractive?

Um, I would say, probably like my stomach is the one thing that makes me unattractive. Because it's not small, for somebody my height, short, should have a small stomach, and like that is what I am trying to work toward, and like when I go to the gym that is what I am trying to focus on becoming, small in the stomach.

6

Okay, do you do these things, like exercising and eating and stuff, is it in any way, would you say, to be attractive to others?

Oh um ... I think at this point, definitely, surely who doesn't? But I think in the long run it's just to be healthy, 'cause I don't want to grow up and not have these habits, because it's going to be harder and harder to get into it. But right now, of course. Like you just want to look good for yourself and for others.

I just want to keep my body toned, it's not so much losing weight, I just want to keep the body image as it is, because right now, as we said before, I'm pretty comfortable what it looks like, so I don't want to change. Um, and I think it has to do with looking good for others, and also it's a confidence issue, when you are happy with the way you look, it's easy to be confident.

2

Where do you think that comes from?

Um ... I would say, a lot of it is compliments. Like, the good things would probably be complimented on by people, I mean like if someone says "oh your hair looks really nice today" you're like, "oh, I do have good hair!" like, and then you like start to notice it. If someone compliments your smile, like, you notice it, and you're like "oh I guess it does look nice," especially if it's something that more than one person, like multiple people saying it's nice, you start to feel like its true.

13

Why don't you like being short?

Because I think like I could, I don't know, sometimes I feel like tall people just look good in some clothes that I could like never pull off, you know? Like even in capris sometimes I'm like "I'm too short for capris!" I just wish I had long, slender legs, I guess.

18

Now for you personally, do you think that you eat healthy and you go to the gym to, do you think part of it is basically to be attractive to others?

Umm, I think it's a nice benefit, and I think that, I think that, I'm trying to, I enjoy it so I don't really think about it in that way, but I think that, well I guess when I go home, if it's snowing out, and I don't have a gym to go to, I don't go exercising I just watch what I eat more. So I guess you could kind of count that as like worrying what I look like, but at the same time, I like doing those things for me to be healthy. And I mean I still, you like being thin, I do it to stay in shape and to look decent, but I think there are other factors as well.

10

Do you feel that for girls on campus that there's pressure to dress a certain way?

Freshmen? Um, sometimes, I mean, I think that everyone wants to look hot you know and everyone wants to like, yeah, like go out, when we go out in the courts and party everyone wants to look like hot and you know, feel wanted and stuff, but I don't know, but most of my friends don't care how they look, we're beyond that, you know? So, there are two sides to it definitely.

8

What do you think constitutes a cute girl?

Um, hmm, someone who's put together, someone who had like a pretty distinct clique of other cute girls, like uh, I dunno, it's like a phenomenon of youth that did make you cool.

And like that's pretty late I think for a girl, uh, and I did it because, well, when I wasn't wearing bras it was because like I wanted my body to look the way that it is and I wanted to just present my body in the form that it was and I didn't want to pretend to ever, like, other people.

4

Um, well I like to be able to wear clothes and feel like I look good in them, so if I try on an outfit and I don't feel like I look good in it I do not buy it, or, um, the way I look is also important to me, so I go to the gym—and although I don't faithfully go four or five times a week, like I would like to, I try to go three or four times a week, because I like to feel like I can keep my body in check so I do not gain a lot of weight.

So why do you think it's necessary to stay an average weight in order to feel attractive?

Well I think it's important, because first of all it's healthy, and second, it's harder to find a relationship to get into one, I think if you feel like you have a poor body image. So if I feel like I am average, I feel healthy, and I look healthy, I will be more attractive to others, and I will have a better relationship, knowing that I am doing things the right way and staying happy.

15

So how about you, how important is it for you to feel physically attractive to people?

Um, I think there is some level in myself where I want to be attracted to other people but I also want to feel like I don't need to portray any particular image to be attractive to people.

14

So you desire to have skinny thighs?

Yes!

Why?

Um, I don't know. That's a good question! [*Giggle*] I don't know, but I mean guess because that is what is seen as attractive by guys. And who doesn't want to be seen as attractive by guys?

I try to go to the gym 5 days a week and I do 20 minutes on the elliptical and then I do power yoga. That's about it, I mean no, is it power yoga? I think it's power yoga ... abs yoga, it's abs yoga! I do 20 minutes on the elliptical and then I do abs yoga for like 15 minutes, so I don't really go that long, but the fact that, like I do that consistently combined with the fact that I try not to eat like complete crap, combined with the fact that I have the ability to lose the weight I feel like that's enough to get me the image, the body image that I want to have.

So, why do you go to the gym overall?

To stay thin.

So why don't you eat it all the time?

Because it's more important for me, to myself to be thin and to look good than to eat what I like.

Research as Poetry

A Couple Experiences HIV

Cynthia Cannon Poindexter

The two poems presented here as exemplars stem from a qualitative research project and are the result of a process of honing the way I approach respondents' language. In 1996 Pat and Doug (pseudonyms), African American heterosexual lovers, talked to me about the emotional turmoil resulting from Doug's having tested positive for HIV after sharing a syringe with a heroin buddy. Pat was 47 years old and Doug was 51. The one-time, open-ended interview occurred during my dissertation study of older HIV-affected caregivers in Chicago, Illinois (see Poindexter & Linsk, 1999). As I was completing the consent form with Pat, Doug asked for permission to talk to me as well. This resulted in audiotaped comments from them both as they sat in their living room together.

The Process

Generating poetry from research interviews has been an iterative process for me. Although my dissertation was in process, I continually feared that I would not be able to sufficiently give voice to the respondents' stories and not be able to translate their experiences in a way that would be useful and meaningful to readers. I was aware that the respondents were counting on me to tell their stories, but I did not feel that I had the language at that time to express their experiences. At that time, I had not yet learned of the field of narrative studies, James Gee's (1985, 1986, 1991) stanza treatment of qualitative data, Laurel Richardson's (1992, 1994) and Bettina Becker's (1999) research-based poetry, or Prattis's (1985) report of anthropologists who were writing poetry about their fieldwork.

During the data collection, I ran across the idea of crafting a "poem" for each of the participants by reading one line in the Miles and Huberman (1994, p. 110) qualitative methods book. As I did so, I felt relief that I would at least be more satisfied in private if I could craft poetry out of respondents' stories. I decided to include the poems as an appendix in my dissertation, but I never anticipated that the poetry would be read. Several faculty members on my dissertation committee read them, however, and encouraged me to find outlets for this poetry, which led to five of them being published (see Poindexter, 1997a, 1997b). One of these poems was derived from the female respondent presented here, under a different pseudonym (Jen) and in a different formulation.

The process I followed during my dissertation was simpler and less informed than what I do now. As I coded each transcribed interview, I copied phrases, sentences, or paragraphs that seemed to highlight the unique personality or perspective of the respondent and transferred them into another computer document. At the end of that process, I arranged the respondent's phrases into stanzas that seemed to me to best represent him or her. The result was a poem in the actual words of the interviewee. Although I arranged the words in an order that seemed to best represent the narrative flow and the respondent's meaning, no changes—except in sequencing—were made to the actual wording. I was looking for unambiguous phrases, strong statements, eloquent expressions, wording that appealed to me, and portions of narrative that I felt strongly captured the person I had met and interviewed. This method is so reliant on the gut feeling and literary hunches of the researcher that it cannot be replicated. The aesthetic and emotional criteria are very personal.

The next phase of my writing research poetry happened after I accepted a job at Boston University School of Social Work and interviewed more HIV-affected caregivers. I returned to this method of data re-presentation because of my own emotional connection with the material. The poems seemed to me to be embedded in the stories, just as the stories were embedded in the interviews, and when I extracted them I felt a deeper sense of empathy and resonance with the caregivers' experiences. Also at Boston University I met Dr. Catherine Kohler Riessman and became aware of narrative studies (Riessman, 1993). When she realized that I had produced some research poetry, she introduced me to Laurel Richardson's research poetry and James Gee's work attending to the architecture of speech, arranging utterances into lines, stanzas, and parts.

Using Gee's method, I retranscribed portions of interviews repeatedly, dividing utterances into idea units, lines, and stanzas and attending to respondents' sequencing, pace, tone, and phrasing. Now re-presenting data in Gee's format for presentations and manuscripts, I wanted to use it to improve my method of crafting poetry as well. Instead of starting with rough transcripts, I started with interview excerpts that I had transcribed with emphasis and pauses noted. I still engaged in the "diamond-cutting" activity of carving away all but the phrases and stanzas that seemed most evocative in emotion and clarity, but I did not change the order that the text excerpts appeared in the interview. The result of this more deliberate process is, I hope, the respondents' experiences in a coherent, abridged form, acknowledging their expressions and words. I wish for this treatment of text to render stories into a core narrative, spotlighting ambiguity and highlighting the simplicity and power of the respondents' worlds and words.

The Poems

Doug's poem ("I've Been Knocked Down, but I Haven't Been Knocked Out") is derived from a long narrative concerning the process of testing positive for HIV. He had been physically ill and feared he had HIV because he had shared a syringe one day when he was suffering intensely from heroin withdrawal. He sees this infection incident as a one-time mistake ("Bap! And there it was."). He also expresses hope that if he takes care of his health, he will live long and be alive for the cure. He offers philosophical guidelines in the form of metaphors ("I've been knocked down, but I haven't been knocked out") that illustrate the determination and resilience that help him to cope.

Pat's poem ("Lessons Learned Hard Are Best Learned") comes from her narrative regarding her struggle to accept Doug's HIV infection and the way he acquired it. She uses forceful words such as *snapped* and *tumbled* to express the extent of her emotional turmoil and expresses sadness at the disruption of their sexual relationship and her fear of becoming infected. She is articulate about her anger at him, outraged that poor people are not as able to access treatments, fear and grief about his life being in danger, and hope that if he lives well he will live to see the cure. She too expresses a resilient philosophy in the midst of her laments: "Lessons learned hard are best learned."

Some notes on language are appropriate before presenting the poems. When Doug talks about his "stuff," he means the paraphernalia he used to inject heroin. When he says "sick," he means the symptoms of heroin withdrawal. Also in these poems, vocal emphasis is indicated by *ITALI-CIZED CAPS.*

I've Been Knocked Down, but I Haven't Been Knocked Out

I just *KNEW*
    I had the chance
        that I had HIV.
Before the doctor told me that I was positive,
I knew.

I can tell you the day I got infected.
I always used to use my *OWN* stuff.
I *NEVER* used anybody else's stuff *EXCEPT* this time.
This day,
    this particular day,
        I was very vulnerable.
        And this guy, I used his stuff!
I was feeling so frantic,
    that I used his stuff.
The guy was infected.
That was it.
This one time,
    only once,
        ONCE!
I used his stuff.
    Bap!
        And there it was.

We kept saying,
    "man, we're going to catch it,
        we gonna catch it."
But you know,
    when you use,
        when the sick is on,
            that's the last thing on your mind.

I feel like,
    if I take my medicine,
        try to take it everyday.
and if I live right,
    maybe I'll make it.

I've always been a healthy person.
I feel like I've got a great *CHANCE*.
If I look at it negative,
    I'll fade away,
So I just look at the *GOOD* side.
    I'm *STILL* here.
I've been *KNOCKED* down,
    but I haven't been knocked *OUT*.
I'm going to make it.

Nothing that's worth anything comes *EASY*.
    It always comes *HARD*.
        You have to work at it.

I don't take it lightly.
    I just say, "well, I got it,"
        I live day by day
            and pray to god that people find a cure.

Lessons Learned Hard
Are Best Learned

I *TOOK* him to family clinic,
While he was in*SIDE,*
I was reading the *BIBLE* in the car
and I was like,
    "God *PLEASE* don't let him be *SICK*."
Doing that, I could hear God:
    "it's too *LATE* for this prayer,
        he already *HAS* it."

When we first learned about it—
    Snapped *ME*.
It's the worst thing that ever happened to me.
My whole *WORLD* was tumbled,

and I just *KNEW* I wasn't gonna be able to regroup.
I just *HURT* so *MUCH.*
    I *CRIED* for a year.
'Cause I just couldn't believe this *HAP*pened!
I mean, not to *US, YOU* know.
    We was in *LOVE.*

We can't have *SEX* the way we *HAD* it.
We don't *HAVE* sex the way we used to.
I don't *DESIRE* it, it's *SCARY.*

All I could think about was he had a virus that could *KILL* him
and if I had *SEX* with him I was gonna die *WITH* him.
I was totally stressed out!
    I was *TERR*ified
        I was *HURT*
           I was *CRUSHED.*

I'm *MAD* at him.
    I'm *STILL* mad at him.
I can't believe he *DID* this to us, you know?
    And he's sorry,
        and I know he's sorry,
           but sorry don't make it right.
             Sorry can't *FIX THIS.*

If you *POOR* and *BLACK* and don't have any *MONEY*
    you can't afford the medication.
So, since we *DON'T* have the money,
    we have to have the *FAITH.*
It's a shame when you have to learn all lessons the *HARD* way.
Lessons learned *HARD* are best learned.
    That's the way we feel.

One thing I believe
    from the bottom of my *SOUL*
and that's that you can die from a broken heart.
He's my *EVERY*thing.
And *AS* you can see, I can't talk about it *LONG* without crying.

I give *OFF* this air that I'm so strong,
    but *AIDS* will knock you to your knees.

The thought of the person that *YOU* love more than anything in the
world—
It broke me all the way down to my knees.

He looks pretty *WELL* for a person that has *AIDS*.
So I *TRY* not to deal with it.
I just try to deal with the fact that he *LOOK* healthy,
what can I do to *KEEP* him lookin healthy,
showing him I *LOVE* him,
don't let him see that I'm *WORRIED*.
I think that, if he takes his medicine,
if I feed him *WELL,*
that he can over*COME* this,
and maybe one day they'll find a *CURE*.

Conclusions

Doug and Pat are separate people with different health statuses and
divergent perspectives. Doug is focused on his own strength, and Pat is
focused on her own grief. Yet they share rhetoric to a remarkable degree.
They both talk about Doug's taking care of himself so he can live until the
cure. They both acknowledge that they cannot reconcile her anger and
lack of understanding about his sharing a syringe. They both attribute
daily functioning to faith in God. And they both use the word *hard* to
express their life philosophy. Doug declares, "Nothing that's worth anything comes easy. It always comes hard." And Pat says, "Lessons learned
hard are best learned."

Poetry formed from respondents' words, although perhaps not
appropriate for re-presenting data in a scholarly report, is nevertheless a
form that may be of use in classes and training sessions. Several times I
have used poetry crafted from research interviews to end presentations
and workshops, as well as in conference poster sessions, and have found
that listeners and readers tend to be moved by their simplicity and power.
As Richardson (1993) stated, the intent of the research poem is both aesthetic and empathic: It can communicate the respondent's emotional
world effectively and efficiently. In developing a poem, the researcher
selects talk and reforms it into a nontraditional re-presentation. The
resulting poem may bring points to the fore, clarify and make the account
more compelling, create a different effect, engage the reader and listener,
and tell us something about lived experience that we did not previously
understand.

Qualitative researchers struggling to use their work for advocacy and for raising awareness may want to experiment with poetic representations. The disadvantage of using research poetry is that its usefulness as a form of data re-presentation is debated and controversial. Although there are accepted norms and standards for other methods of presenting data, there are none for research poetry. Do we evaluate them by artistic or scientific means? Do we judge them because we better understand a type of situation or a group of people or because we more fully understand one particular person? Perhaps the most applicable standard is whether they further empathy and/or understanding. The advantage of research poetry may be that core narratives and strong emotions can be communicated with an economy of words. Poems perhaps facilitate teaching through the power of language.

References

Becker, B. (1999). Narratives of pain in later life and conventions of storytelling. *Journal of Aging Studies, 13*(1), 73–87.

Gee, J. (1985). The narrativization of experience in the oral style. *Journal of Education, 167*(1), 9–35.

Gee, J. (1986). Units in the production of narrative discourse. *Discourse Processes, 9*(4), 391–422.

Gee, J. (1991). A linguistic approach to narrative. *Journal of Narrative and Life History, 1*(1), 15–39.

Miles, M. B., & Huberman, A. M. (1994). *Qualitative data analysis* (2nd ed.). Thousand Oaks, CA: Sage.

Poindexter, C. C. (1997a, December). Ms. Carol and Ms. Dorothy (research poetry). *Affilia: Journal of Women and Social Work, 12*(4), 486–489.

Poindexter, C. C. (1997b). Poetry as data analysis: Listening to the narratives of older minority HIV-affected caregivers. *Reflections: Narratives of Professional Helping, 4*(3), 22–25.

Poindexter, C. C., & Linsk, N. (1999). HIV-related stigma in a sample of HIV-affected older female African-American caregivers. *Social Work, 44*(1), 46–61.

Prattis, J. I. (Ed). (1985). *Reflections: The anthropological muse.* Washington, DC: American Anthropological Association.

Richardson, L. (1992). The consequences of poetic representation: Writing the other, rewriting the self. In C. Ellis & M. G. Flaherty (Eds.), *Investigating subjectivity: Research on lived experience* (pp. 125–137). Newbury Park, CA: Sage.

Richardson, L. (1993). Poetics, dramatics, and transgressive validity: The case of the skipped line. *Sociological Quarterly, 34*(4), 695–710.

Richardson, L. (1994). Nine poems: Marriage and the family. *Journal of Contemporary Ethnography, 23*(1), 3–13.

Riessman, C. K. (1993). *Narrative analysis.* Newbury Park, CA: Sage.

CHAPTER 4

◝◟◞◜

Music and Qualitative Research

> Our engagement as musicians with the fluidity of sound and
> music, I argue, can sensitize us to the fluidity of personal and
> cultural experience, the heart of qualitative research.
> —LIORA BRESLER (2005, p. 170)

Louis Armstrong famously noted that, as jazz musicians, "what we play
is life." Similarly, literary giant Leo Tolstoy professed, "Music is the short-
hand of emotion." Although the turn to music in social research may
seem suspect to some, if society were compared to a living body, a comparison that is frequently made, one could argue music would be flow-
ing through its veins. The use of music in social research methodologies
can be viewed less as an experiment and more as a *realization.* In fact,
music-based methods can help researchers access, illuminate, describe,
and explain that which is often rendered invisible by traditional research
practices. As Aldous Huxley said, "After silence, that which comes near-
est to expressing the inexpressible is music."

Popularly termed "the universal language," music is innately social,
a penetrating part of every culture. Although now (re)emerging as part
of arts-based methods of social inquiry across the disciplines, music has
long been a part of social research, with roots in anthropological studies of folklore as well as research in music education. From a social science perspective music can be many things (simultaneously), including
a commodity, an ideological text, a political tool, a resistive tool, and an
integral component of cultural rituals and daily social life.

Music can be defined in many ways, particularly when thinking cross-
culturally, so my suggestions for how to define or conceptualize music are

inherently limited. Nevertheless, music is generally considered to be the art of arranging sounds into a continuous and unified composition with dimensions that typically include rhythm and melody (*en.wikipedia.org/ wiki/definition_of_music*). Music generally refers to sounds with distinct pitches that are arranged into melodies and organized into patterns of rhythm; songs in many genres also include lyrics, often arranged as a narrative with bridges and repeating choruses. In Western culture there are norms for creating harmony that are also integral to the making of music. Music also has a symbolic system or language through which it is written. As Robert Walker (1992) explains, the visual, symbolic forms "act as mnemonics for the physical actions necessary in the production of musical or spoken sounds" (p. 344). As with any other discipline, music education has a unique epistemology and structure as well as specialized jargon (Richardson & Whitaker, 1992, p. 549).

Songs and musical scores are conceived for many purposes, including the evocation of emotion, the creation of beauty, and the growth of the individual artist, and it is also a part of many cultural rituals. Music is able to *connect* people through emotional evocation that in certain contexts may transcend language, economic, and other social barriers. Poet Robert Browning expressed this sentiment best: "Who hears music, feels his solitude peopled at once."

Despite its presumed universality, as with other arts music is a cultural product imprinted with material and symbolic aspects of its point of production as well as the musical conventions prevalent in that time and place. Music is created in cultural and historical contexts and thus varies across time and space. Although popularly thought of as "a universal language," music only unites people within certain contexts and can also identify differences across cultures and ethnicities and comment on those differences (Elliott, 1989; Jordan, 1992).

Moreover, philosophers have posited that music is intrinsically social in ways that extend beyond its status as a socially constructed art form. Philosopher Theodor Adorno and economist Jacques Attali, each influenced by Karl Marx's analysis of capitalism, theorized about the social importance of music long before music was taken seriously in the social sciences. For Adorno, who (influenced by Marx) considered the political economy of music, saw music not as an add-on to human experience, but rather as a significant force in shaping consciousness. In Adorno's (1984) work not all music has the same value. Popular music, driven by a market economy, creates conformity, passivity, and thus contributes to "false consciousness." On the other end of the spectrum, some other kinds of music can subvert and resist stereotypical, complacent group thinking (false consciousness), and therefore music has resistive capabilities that can propel altered social consciousness and transgress the dominant order.

Attali (1985) examined the implication of music in relations of power, particularly economic and political power. Like Adorno, Attali analyzed music as an agent of social control with insidious workings in the execution and maintenance of social power, far more than the popular perception of music as entertainment would suggest.

In addition, music is a fluid art form that bears similarities to the fluidity of lived experience (Bresler, 2005, p. 170). For example, *improvisation* is often critical to the making of music, and this practice involves a responsiveness to unexpected situations that is true of both social life and our study of it, particularly when using qualitative approaches (Bresler, 2005, p. 174). With respect to qualitative research, an openness, flexibility, and malleability on the part of the researcher is central to knowledge-building and dealing with the unpredictable elements of ethnographic field sites as well as the fluid nature of open-ended interviews (Bresler, 2005, p. 175). In this regard, Bresler notes that both music and social research can be "grounded within a paradigm of fluidity" (2005, p. 174). The fluidity of music is also linked to the performative aspect of the art, discussed in greater depth later. For now it is important to understand that music is a "happening" that comes to be via performance (Stubley, 1995, p. 62), thus differing from written or visual art. In this book music is placed between the chapters on poetry and performance because poetry is a lyrical textual form and music is a performance-based medium.

As Jacques Attali suggested, sound and "noise" more generally are virtually a constant component of social life, far more insidious in the daily shaping of experience than we might realize. More specifically, music is used for many purposes and incorporated into many parts of a society. For example, music is often a part of religious or spiritual rituals and practices, ceremonies related to weddings or funerals, as well as educational markers such as graduation, popular entertainment, or leisure time activities, and a great many other components of culture. In addition, this medium communicates a variety of information to the society: providing insight into particular historical periods, power relations, social struggles or movements, social or political resistance, and personal or collective experience related to any number of characteristics or circumstances (e.g., racial or gender inequality, the experience of war, violence, sexuality, euphoria or pain from drug use, or extreme ecstasy and pleasure). The particular power of music as a vehicle of information sharing in these and other ways is now being harnessed by qualitative researchers who are creating research methodologies that use music as a model for data analysis and interpretation as well as a representational form that may be textual or performance-based.

Given the narrative capabilities of lyrical songs, in many cultures music is viewed as a major form of storytelling. For example, in Korea the performative art form *P'ansori* combines singing and storytelling and is believed to reveal social and political elements of Korean culture (Grossberg, 2005). The narrative capabilities of music are central to the current transformation of music into a representational form for social research.

Multiculturalism, Hybridity, and Ethnomusicology

Over the past three decades music education has been one locus of attention for larger movements in the United States toward multiculturalism and pluralism (Jordan, 1992, p. 735). However, an interest in music from different cultures has been a part of music education long before the multiculturalism movements of the past few decades (Anderson, 1974; Jordan, 1992). Music, always produced by social actors situated in groups, can offer many insights into the peoples and cultures that produce it, including identity issues and points of similarity and difference across ethnicities. There are many ways that culturally diverse music can, and has been, included in public education. Typically, music from other cultures has been included in American music education, but this music has been exoticized and relegated to visitor status within the music curriculum. In the context of America's culturally pluralistic society, we might conceive of a music education curriculum that includes music from diverse cultures with the intent of cultivating a "world perspective" as opposed to including various music but using Western standards as the benchmark by which they are judged and thus privileging one musical tradition over others (something that has already occurred under the rubric of multicultural music education) (Jordan, 1992). Looking at the role of world music in American education—and its relationship to larger issues pertaining to diversity, voice, and cultural representation—can provide many insights into social phenomena while raising questions such as: What might a world music curriculum consist of, and how would it be organized? What might it teach students about anthropology, globalization, development, ethnicity, diversity, democracy, nationalism, and, of course, different musical systems from a music perspective?

From a social science perspective an extension of considering the relationship between music and multiculturalism is examining music as a locus of hybridity—a space in which different elements, often from different cultures, times, or genres, merge to create something new. Hybridity scholars refer to this as a "third space" (Bhabha, 1993) that emerges when aspects of different cultures merge, opening a new site for the production and negotiation of culture. The term *third space* does not derive from an additive model but rather from the opening of a space where something new develops. The opportunity and need to investigate musical hybrids has increased exponentially with globalization and the multidirectional cultural exchange it has fostered. In this regard, the turn to music as an object of social inquiry allows researchers interested in cultural aspects of globalization a data source in which processes of hybridization are embedded. Because hybrid music always requires a mixing of sounds, genres, or cultures, there is great potential to study collective identity struggles and negotiations via this medium.[1] For the purpose of this exploration, I suggest that the surge in hybridity in music parallels the emergence of hybrid arts-based methods that rely on musical forms. In other words, the hybridity we are seeing in music creation is also found in the creation of music-based research methods. Moreover, hybrid musical forms may open up a space to further develop the music-based methods reviewed later in this chapter, where, for example, international research collaborations may develop as sound files are exchanged over the Internet or interview data representation incorporates music or sound elements from participants' cultures.

Within the study of music itself, *ethnomusicology* is a disciplinary hybrid with roots in both anthropology and musicology. Ethnomusicology involves the study of music in other cultures. In musicology, studies often involve comparing musical systems cross-culturally (Bresler & Stake, 1992, p. 80). In anthropology, studies aim to understand the music of a culture in the context of that culture and human interaction therein (Bresler & Stake, 1992, p. 80). As with other forms of ethnography, these studies typically occur in natural settings, where researchers immerse themselves in the culture in an effort to understand music *within* the larger cultural context (Bresler & Stake, 1992, p. 80). Nicole Carrigan (2003) has conducted studies using this method and explains that when going from one musical culture to another, social researchers must consider three dimensions of how music fits into the culture: the conceptual, the contextual, and the circumstantial (p. 42). Furthermore, citing Stobin and Titon (1992), she advocates four categories for developing a cross-cultural perspective: (1) ideas about music, (2) social organization of music, (3) repertoires of music, and (4) material culture of music.

Music as a Model for Qualitative Research

Although music (and dance) remain the least-explored art forms with respect to arts-based methods, more frequently serving as subjects of social inquiry rather than tools through which to conduct social research, in recent years exciting methodological innovations have begun to emerge. These emergent practices are on the cutting edge of arts-based research and qualitative methods more broadly. In this chapter I review three innovations: (1) music as a model of qualitative research, (2) musical portraiture, and (3) performance collage. (The latter two are music-based methods of analysis, interpretation, and representation.) It is in the discussion the two music-based research methods that the possibilities of "music as a model" come into existence and are pushed beyond theoretical constructs.

Liora Bresler (2005) has been at the forefront of theorizing about the relationship between music and qualitative research, and more specifically how music can help sensitize qualitative researchers to the fluidity of social life and bring greater attention to many of the issues they are already interested in. Western culture is considered a "visual culture." In this context, Bresler explains people are sight-driven and therefore researchers have created methodologies that are also sight-based, such as constructing knowledge via visual observation. As all qualitative researchers know, however, in ethnographic and interview research *hearing* is integral to the knowledge-building process, and skills associated with music can help researchers build their listening skills with great depth and intricacy. Later in this chapter I suggest that music can help us access and shed light on parts of social experience that other textual or visual forms may fail to capture. Bresler argues that by adopting "musical lenses" or "musical sensitivities" when engaged in qualitative research, the researcher may be able to access dimensions of the subject and research process that would otherwise remain untapped (pp. 170–171).

Bresler (2005) offers a model built from metaphors in which all formal dimensions of music can be adapted to highlight dimensions of social experience that may not be fully attended to in traditional qualitative research projects. These dimensions of music include: form, rhythm, dynamics, timbre, melody, polyphony, and harmony. A new conceptualization and application of these aspects of music can assist researchers in the three major techniques associated with qualitative research, which are, in general terms, perception, conceptualization, and communication (p. 172). Moreover, I suggest that researchers who conduct ethnographic and interview studies think about how Bresler's categories could be implemented as a coding strategy and/or as a framework for structuring the written representation of research findings.

- How can some of these dimensions of music be employed to enhance qualitative research methodologies? How can they build effective listening skills? How can they be adapted as a coding strategy or framework for representation?

Form speaks to the organization of music. In other words, form refers to how the parts and whole are conceived as well as how variation, unity, and repetition are organized. Bresler (2005) notes that form, in these ways, is also integral to social life and our writings about it, in which we must negotiate how the parts of a person's story fit together; where variation and repetition can occur to impart meaning; and how to employ conventions such as organizing our data into stories with beginnings, middles, and ends (p. 172). Researchers can use music to contemplate the importance of form in life and research—perhaps the transcendental quality of music will inject new awareness into this process and help the researcher to reconsider the relations of parts within the whole. As a result, conventions of writing up research findings might be unsettled as researchers adapt a music-based template to their writing format.

There are also several aspects of music that attend to how meaning is communicated and can offer qualitative researchers lenses through which to view how their participants create and communicate meaning. These dimensions focus on patterns, pace, tone, inflection, and texture. *Rhythm* refers to temporal patterns (tempo being pace) and to the relationships between tempi (Bresler, 2005, p. 173). Attention to rhythm helps shape how researchers communicate knowledge; for example, this is clear in the way researchers construct conference presentations and other public talks. *Dynamics* has to do with how "loudness" and "softness" are perceived differently, depending on the context. For example, the same sound may be perceived as louder or softer based solely on what it follows, and how loud or soft that preceding note is. Bresler writes, "Silence feels different just before the music starts, as compared to immediately following a climax, or as closure" (p. 173). Dynamics are also active in social interactions shaping "anticipation, tension, confrontations, resolutions" (p. 173).

Next, researchers can consider *timbre*. This concept refers to the musical color, inflection, and tone that are all integral to how meaning is conveyed. This dimension may be particularly important to qualitative researchers engaged in interactive research methods such as in-depth interviews, focus group interviews, oral histories, and ethnography, all of which require an acute attention not just to *what* participants say but also to *how* they say it, and how communication styles also impart meaning. Researchers dealing with disenfranchised or disempowered populations; those working from feminist and other critical perspectives; as well as those interested in accessing the subjugated knowledges of women, people of color, homosexuals, and others forced to the margins of the society may find an attention to "timbres" particularly useful. Bresler notes that timbres can offer a window onto gender and race differences as well as individual differences (2005, p. 173).

Polyphony, in musical composition, creates texture through simultaneous lines of sound as well as through the interrelation of the lines. This structural concept bears directly on the fluid nature of social life, which "consists of simultaneously multiple voices, sometimes silent, always present—thinking, interacting, experiencing, creating the texture of life" (Bresler, 2005, p. 174). Moreover, "texture creates and enables harmony" (p. 174). This is both a wonderful metaphor for the study of difference and diversity and a way of tuning researchers in to those aspects of social life wherein texture and harmony emerge. In this regard, Bresler notes, "As researchers, we attend to the dissonances and consonances of social life, often appreciating the interplay between dissonant moments and their resolutions or lack of" (p. 174). This approach may be particularly appealing to feminist researchers as well as to qualitative researchers studying race, sexuality, and related topics.

Finally, *melody* refers to the "plotline," including what emotions and climaxes are built into the plot, such as anticipation or drama (Bresler & Stake, 1992, p. 84). Researchers can apply this concept during their interpretation and analysis of interview or focus-group data. Moreover, as researchers write up their findings they can pay attention to the melodic structure of their writing, considering how they place emphasis and how different audiences might receive the work. Furthermore, researchers interested in preserving their respondents' voices (both words and tonal dimensions) can write in a melodic structure that mirrors their participants' telling of their own stories.

The categories offered by Bresler could be applied to the data collection phase of qualitative research (e.g., via listening techniques), during analysis and interpretation (serving as a method for organizing and coding field notes or interview transcripts), and as a format for representation. These approaches could thus be used in conjunction with more traditional qualitative methods or could service projects that employ less conventional methods such as autoethnography or multivocal autoethnography (see Davis & Ellis, 2008).

- How can Bresler's categories be put into action? What additional methodological issues require attention? How can these metaphors be pushed further to extend the possibilities of arts-based research?

Portraiture, Sonic Analysis, and Performance Collage: Innovative Music-Based Research Methods

An exciting adaptation and clear extension of using music as a mode for qualitative research comes from Terry Jenoure's (2002) work "Sweeping the Temple," in which she develops two music-based research methods. The first, which she refers to as *musical portraiture*, is the process of coding data using musical structures, with the result being *sonic narratives* she likens to "jazz riffs." The latter method, *performance collage*, refers to the process of musically coding and writing up data culminating in a musical performance. Although she titles her two music-based methods portraiture and performance collage, I suggest that researchers working with these and related approaches in the future might also consider the terms "sonic interpretation schema," "multidimensional sonic performance," "musical collage," "musical tapestry," "sonic research writing," and "sonic narrative writing."

As with many researchers at the cutting edge of arts-based research, Jenoure's methods innovation developed when traditional methods left a project feeling "unfinished." The project also emerged at a complex personal and professional intersection. Jenoure is a social scholar and musician who was working on a book about African American artists who teach at historically white colleges. During this time her best friend and artistic collaborator of 20 years, Patti, a dancer, was diagnosed with breast cancer. Patti was one of the interviewees for the book and even agreed to videotape one interview session in the latter stages of her cancer battle. Patti fought her illness for 2 years and died. Jenoure finished the book that featured her dear friend as one of four "portraits" developed out of the interview data.

The portrait method that Jenoure employed in the book emerged out of an artistic approach to analysis, interpretation, and writing, one that drew on her musical and research skills. During the process of reviewing the data Jenoure, in a manner she describes as virtually "automatic," began aligning particular kinds of comments. Although this may seem unremarkable to qualitative researchers, the artist part of Jenoure saw the musicality in this process. She writes:

> I realized that what I had was a series of short conversations. I was composing sound again. I was making songs and I could hear them in my head and it felt perfect. Best of all, I felt more like myself. ... (2002, p. 77)

Using this emerging methodology Jenoure created "characters" out of the interview data and paid attention to such issues as tension, textures, colors, rhythms, brightness, pauses, and accelerations (2002, p. 77). These aspects of music extended far beyond the metaphors and conceptual categories delineated by Bresler and became a way of *organizing* and *writing* the data into textual pieces that embody musicality. Through this process she created "hushes," "screams," "drum rolls," and "cymbal crashes" (p. 77).

As is often the case when working with an innovative methodology, unexpected issues can spring forth during the process. In this instance, Jenoure engaged in extensive contemplation regarding the ethical implications of her work. The sonic form her analysis was producing made her respondents at times appear as if in conversation, which had not actually occurred. Comfortable that she had not altered anyone's words, she forged ahead and even added her own voice into the mix in the role of interviewer.

This entire analytical process resulted in pieces that Jenoure, borrowing from the language of jazz improvisation, termed "riffs," and were incorporated into the book (2002, p. 78). She notes that in jazz, riffs are used to "punctuate a musical idea"; with this conceptual frame in place, the vibrant "riffs" were woven throughout the book.

Despite the successful incorporation of musicality into her work, the completion of the original project coupled with the devastating loss of her friend left Jenoure feeling unsatisfied. With respect to Patti, she felt that her story and their story of friendship and collaboration had not been fully told in the monograph. In addition, the subject of her book—interviews with people who had balanced their scholarly and artistic lives—made Jenoure feel like an "outsider" to her own project, particularly on the heels of 2 years without performing (so that she could complete the book). The musical element of her work still placed her in the role of "researcher" and, as many researchers who take on arts-based research do, she retained an artist identity that was unfulfilled. Jenoure writes:

> My artist-self felt the way I always do when I've gone through long, dry spells of musical celibacy, then gone to hear my colleagues in concert; me: stiff, tense, and awkward, them: on stage, illuminated in their spirit bodies, wings and all. In those moments, I'm sad, overjoyed, frustrated, inspired, depressed, exuberant, and confused, all at the same time. (2002, p. 76)

Jenoure's candor in this area is, I think, deeply generous and vitally important. Many researchers who work with arts-based methods also embody an artistic identity. Traditional, legitimized scientific practices, including conventional approaches to qualitative research, often force artist-researchers to disavow a part of their identity in order to produce publishable work and meet tenure, promotion, and funding criteria. As arts-based methods expand the borders of what constitutes legitimate science, researchers who struggle to balance their academic and artistic lives may have an easier time. Beyond Jenoure's desire to perform again, the absence of a performance element left a dimension of the work *underrealized*. She felt compelled to integrate the different parts of her life and complete this work, and Patti's unfinished story provided the material.

Jenoure returned to the data from Patti as well as her own auto-ethnographic data and found that she had two main groups of data: Patti's stories and her own poems. From the data Jenoure composed a musical performance using taped and live excerpts—the mixing of the two intended to create "depth" and "reverberation." Spoken prose was relegated to the taped segments while poems were sung live. Repetitive phrases were also employed to shape rhythm.

Jenoure's research was highly successful relative to her goals. She effectively developed two music-based methods: one textual and one performance-based. In terms of the former, the sonic portraiture Jenoure created has the potential to move forward not only music-based methods innovations but also our understanding and execution of narrative analysis. The latter method suggests an additional embodied method of (re)presentation in addition to the dramatic and dance forms reviewed in the next two chapters.

Music as Data:
Possibilities for Merging
Musical Data and Music-Based Methods

The use of music as a source of data in social research derives from the idea that music is a cultural text, and, as with other cultural texts, by examining music we can investigate a range of questions about the culture in which the text was produced. Music can also be classified as an *object* that is open to inquiry (Morrison, 1992). Moreover, it is a text in which ideology is embedded (Holman Jones, 2002). Music in its textual or printed form is commonly studied via content analysis, in which musical notations are rendered as symbolic data (Casey, 1992, p. 121).

There is also a resistive or political potential to music that may or may not be activated within different performance or listening contexts. For decades many scholars across the disciplines have understood the vital role music has played in African American social historical experiences and our understanding of them as a form of political resistance, a coping strategy for dealing with racism, entertainment, a cultural tracking system, a vehicle for success in a racist society, and many other purposes.

Warrick Carter (1973) researched the presence of music, among other art forms, in black studies programs at colleges and universities in the United States. His research hinged on his contention that music is an important source of information about black culture. This is particularly salient because African Americans have been excluded from the production of other aspects of American society, or their contributions have been marginalized and relegated to the dustbins of social history. By examining the music black Americans have created at different historical moments, such as jazz, blues, soul, rap, and hip-hop, as well as their participation in predominantly white musical genres such as rock, classical, and opera, students can learn about social struggles and experiences of inequality, despair, and hope that developed from their lived experiences in a racist society. Furthermore, students can explore how music has served as a vehicle for sharing these experiences and feelings, as well as communicating a range of ideas about the experiences and identity struggles of black Americans during various historical moments. By using music as a part of the representation of research results, social action researchers can try to promote understanding of issues of inequality while also inspiring audiences to work toward eradicating such issues.

More than three decades ago Carter posited that music could offer great insight into black history as well as the multiple emotional experiences of black Americans at different times and in different contexts. Carter wrote:

> It seems that it has been very easy for organizers of Black Studies programs to forget the importance of music in the struggle for total freedom. Let me remind you of the extra-musical meanings to be found in the text of both the spirituals and the blues. In addition, music has been the "safety valve" through which many blacks have been able to release their emotions. (1973, p. 148)

Imagine present-day possibilities for a study of this kind, given the recent emergence of music-based methods of analysis and representation. For example, consider an interview project with Hurricane Katrina survivors

in New Orleans who formerly worked in the jazz club scene. Imagine analyzing and interpreting the interview transcripts employing the method
Jenoure used in "Sweeping the Temple": the interview transcripts woven
together as a sonic conversation perhaps filled in and punctuated not
by the researcher's voice, as in the case of Jenoure's research, but rather
punctuated with live or recorded jazz music. Depending on the research
purpose and context, audio news coverage from the event aftermath may
be incorporated into the musical collage as well. The possibilities are
open.

Embodiment and the Mind–Body Dichotomy

The increase in social scientific research projects exploring music (and
dance) and creating music-based methods innovations is linked to overall increases in studies of embodiment, the body, and bodily experience
(see Grosz, 1994; Merleau-Ponty, 1962; Pillow, 2001; Spry, 2001) as well
as to feminists and others who continue to dismantle the mind–body
dichotomy (see Bordo, 1993; Butler, 1993; Hesse-Biber, 1996, 2006;
Leavy, Gnong, & Sardi-Ross, 2007; Sprague & Zimmerman, 1993; Wolf,
1991) upon which much traditional social science rests (as discussed
with respect to positivism in Chapter 1). The making of music, inextricably linked to its performance (whether in practice or the formal performance), is a site of embodiment for both the performer and listener. In
this vein, Bresler writes:

> Music is produced by physical movement—the voice or an instrument which
> functions as the extension of the body, where the performer unites with the
> instrument to produce sound ... in performance ... music is experienced,
> not as something given to the body, but as something done through and
> with the body. Sound penetrates us, engaging us on a bodily level in funda-
> mentally different ways than the visual, for example. (2005, pp. 176–177)

Similarly, Stubley notes that audiences do not distinguish between instrument and performer but rather experience them as one (1995, p. 59).
The performative aspect of music is inextricably linked to methodological developments in this area.

In accord with music as an embodied experience, the performing
or making of music exposes, challenges, and dismantles the mind–body
dichotomy in ways that are relevant to social science and particularly the
expansion of the qualitative paradigm. Stubley (1995) goes on to posit
that the unique experience of music blurs our "sensations and percep-

tual boundaries," and that performing music has a spiritual component as "oneness" is experienced (p. 59). Bresler concurs, adding that both the mind and body are actively present as we perceive and interpret music and that this "mind–body presence" is central to qualitative research, in which we constantly send messages to our participants through body language, posture, physical proximity, and so forth. These factors are particularly salient in cross-cultural research or when outsider status is in play (2005, p. 177). Moreover, as researchers try to create a space in which interaction and conversation can occur, we can benefit from attending to the mind–body oneness that occurs in music (p. 177). Furthermore, by using music during the representation stage of research we can affect audience members in new ways, which may again be particularly appealing to social action researchers.

Music as Performance

Although it may be analyzed as a cultural "text" or "object," music is not merely a text or thing: it is *performed* and *heard.* In this respect, music comes to be at the point of articulation, that is, during performance (Rhodes, 1963, p. 198). Similarly, music can be thought of as an event or a "happening," and one that is necessarily singular because no two performances are alike, nor is a particular score or song performed quite the same by different musicians, each with his or her own "musical voice" (Stubley, 1995). In this way, musical performances bear similarities to focus-group interviews, which also provide a "happening" and which, regardless of the degree of structure and control imposed, are never identical (Hesse-Biber & Leavy, 2006). Stubley (1998) explains that musicians search for something beyond the score as they *make* music (p. 93).

In addition, as with poetry, lyrical music utilizes space and breathing to evoke emotional responses. Unlike in poetry, space in music exists during performance. Moreover, space surrounds every musical note, and singers and musicians can manipulate or sculpt these spaces, by elongating them for instance, to produce the desired audience response and, correspondingly, impart meaning. The transformation of musical composition into audible sound thus unleashes its potential to access or reveal emotions as well as to elicit emotional responses from listeners. Jenoure's (2002) use of repetition and rhythm in her sonic writing exemplifies these issues.

The resistive, transcendent, and transformational possibilities of music also come into being through performance, which is another reason why social scientists might be particularly interested in the performative aspect of this and other art forms. Stacy Holman Jones's (2002) research on the emotional and resistive space opened up by torch singing provides an excellent analysis of this facet of music-based research (by torch songs she is referring to formulaic songs of unrequited love performed by female artists such as the hit "Memories," sung by Barbra Streisand). This genre of songs speaks to commonalities many (heterosexual) women may experience as a result of relationship norms related to their gendered location in the social system, although other differences (race, social class, etc.) may come into play. As this research shows, torch songs open up a space of engagement and transcendence at the point of performance.

At the level of "engagement" Holman Jones draws on postcolonial feminism and other critical perspectives to show how, without essentializing women and disavowing difference, the performance of torch songs allows the audience to engage in what is common to their experience as women, thereby building bonds and forging community. Therefore, this is an implicitly *political* form of engagement. In terms of "transcendence," during performance there may be a suspension or tabling of difference (in a certain respect)—a space in which differences are transcended and "common understanding" emerges (2002, p. 748). Alternatively, the space that opens may offer an opportunity for dialogue, an exchange of ideas, and a multiplicity of voices (Conquergood, 1985; Holman Jones, 2002).

Holman Jones also suggests that performance can provide the means for an "oppositional consciousness" that can manifest in many spheres of public life (2002, p. 748). Torch singing involves expressing the suffering of unrequited love as experienced by women, which Holman Jones views as an inherently resistive medium (and act) in which female singers call forth gendered experiences of heterosexual relationships. Torch singers tell their listeners stories so that they may come to new understandings and envision a new "set of possibilities" (p. 739). In light of music-based methodological innovations, it is not hard to imagine how research such as this could be taken to the next level, transforming itself into arts-based research by analyzing and representing the data in sonic form. For example, a multimethod project might combine interviews with women with popular recorded torch songs, written as performance collages. Postperformance interviews could elicit further data for creating portraits.

The political, community-building, and transcendent possibilities associated with the performative dimension of torch singing can be applied and tailored to any number of musical genres in the service of a host of research questions. For instance, consider how African American audience members might experience performances of blues music in a given time and place as well as the spaces such performances might open with respect to transcending differences, building coalitions, and expanding consciousness, which are all preconditions for grassroots social movements. Analyzing and interpreting the data using the musical categories Bresler suggests might thus further create a harmony between the subject and form as well as a synergy between the research purpose and audience, creating a holistic project with social action capabilities. Going further, the data could be written as musical portraiture or made into a musical performance.

Checklist of Considerations

When considering using music in your research, consider the following questions:

✓ What is the purpose of the study and how can music serve as a medium to shed light on this topic?

✓ What is my conception of music? In this study, is music conceptualized as a text, as an object, as a sign system, as a performance, or as some combination of these? Am I interested in the textual form of music, music at the moment of articulation, or both?

✓ What form will the musical data be in? For example, are the data in the form of compositions, scores, and lyrics, or am I interested in the performative, audible aspect of music? In terms of the latter, will live performances be recorded, or will audiotapes be used? Will the physical performance serve as data, or only the music itself?

✓ What is the analysis strategy? For example, will the music alone be analyzed or will data be gathered regarding people's subjective experience of the musical performance via interviews or other methods? In terms of the latter, what do I want to learn from the research participants (e.g., their process of creating meaning out of the music, their identity negotiations, their experiences of resistance or community-building, transcendental qualities of the performance).

✓ If using music as a model for conducting qualitative research, how will I pay attention to dynamics, rhythm, texture, and harmony during my observations and interviews? How will my understanding of form affect my writing process? How will I adapt these principles in order to attend to issues of difference and diversity? What form will my writing/representation take?

Conclusion

As you can see, researchers are broadening their understanding of texts to include music in social research. This allows social researchers a medium through which to readdress research questions explored with more traditional qualitative methods, such as those that pertain to racial and gender inequality, while also opening up a whole range of new research questions relevant to contemporary life. For example, through music researchers can ask timely questions regarding hybrid identities in a shifting global context. In addition, questions that would otherwise remain unasked, such as those that are advancing studies of embodiment, can be explored via music.

Although music has a role in social science—one that has not yet been fully realized—there are limitations to what we can understand via music as well. In the reading that follows this chapter, Norma Daykin provides another perspective on the role of music in the social sciences, arguing both for its importance and limitations while providing empirical examples to illustrate her analysis.

DISCUSSION QUESTIONS AND ACTIVITIES

1. How can music serve as a lens through which to explore hybrid identities and how groups and individuals negotiate these identities? Similarly, how can music help researchers access subjugated voices?

2. What happens at the point when music is articulated? How does the performance of music create and transform the music as well as the audience? What possibilities for social resistance emerge through the performance of music? What does it mean to suggest that making and listening to music are embodied activities?

3. This exercise in the analysis and interpretation of music can be done with a partner or on your own. To begin, select a genre of music (rap, heavy metal, folk music, ballads, etc.) and then sample a preselected number of songs (six to eight songs). Proceed to develop an analysis strategy. Given the genre you have selected, what are you interested in (representations of gender, power, identity, sexuality, romantic love, etc.); if you do not have particular interests with respect to your sample, allow the themes to emerge inductively. Next, try listening to the songs in their entirety while writing memo notes regarding your impressions, themes, keywords, and sounds. Make note of possible similarities and differences between songs. Then proceed to a more systematic analysis by determining the unit of analysis (parts of songs, songs in their entirety, etc.) and developing code categories. Continue with analysis. Finally,

start to develop metacodes (major themes) under which the smaller codes fit. Through this process, pay attention to space, breathing, tonality, emotionality, and so forth, in addition to the sounds and lyrics. This exercise is designed to help you practice careful listening as well as to give you some practical experience analyzing audible data, which includes developing a coding procedure.

4. Take an interview transcript and try to identify the major musical dimensions within the transcript such as timbre, melody, dynamics, and rhythm. Take memo notes that address how this kind of "listening" to the transcript affects your understanding of it

SUGGESTED READINGS

Bowman, W. D. (1998). *Philosophical perspectives on music.* New York: Oxford University Press.

This sophisticated book provides an overview of music and philosophy as well as chapters on many subjects explored from philosophical perspectives on music. The perspectives of Plato, Kant, Hegel, Merleau-Ponty, Clifton, Stubley, Adorno, and Attali are among those covered, as well as contemporary feminist and postmodern perspectives. Although the material is primarily theoretical, as music-based methods innovations continue to emerge, researchers may be influenced by these works as they negotiate the interplay of theoretical and methodological advancement.

Colwell, R. (Ed.). (1992). *Handbook of research on music teaching and learning.* New York: Schirmer Books.

This comprehensive review provides a retrospective and prospective review of the field of music education. Accordingly, chapters identify key traditions, historical shifts, major practices, and the like. This handbook will be particularly useful to researchers in education and music education. Sociologists will find the chapter by Liora Bresler and Robert Stake particularly helpful (part of which provides an excellent review of the main facets of qualitative research in general, suggesting how musical components can be used for methodological innovation).

Leong, S. (Ed.). (2003). *Musicianship in the 21st century: Issues, trends, and possibilities.* Marrickville, NSW, Australia: Southwood Press.

In this collection 25 internationally diverse scholars from different disciplines provide essays on a range of issues pertinent to the study of musicianship.

SUGGESTED WEBSITES AND JOURNALS

Journal of Aesthetic Education
    www.press.uillinois.edu/journals/jae.html

    Journal of Aesthetic Education is a peer-reviewed journal that publishes articles from a variety of viewpoints, including philosophical aesthetics education, communications media, and environmental aesthetics.

Popular Music and Society
    www.tandf.co.uk/journals/titles/03007766.html

    Popular Music and Society is a peer-reviewed journal that publishes reviews and articles about various music genres from a social or historical perspective. Articles can be theoretical or empirical. This is an excellent source for sociologists as well as scholars working from a cultural studies background.

Research Studies in Music Education
    www.rsme.callaway.uwa.edu.au/home

    Research Studies in Music Education is a peer-reviewed journal that publishes articles about the research methodologies used in music education. This journal is particularly well suited to researchers with a music education background, as well as to methodologists.

Music Education Research
    www.tandf.co.uk/journals/titles/14613808.asp

    Music Education Research is a peer-reviewed journal that publishes articles in all areas of music education. A philosophical, sociological, or comparative study, or a psychological perspective in analyzing research and methodological issues is encouraged for submitters.

Ethnomusicology
    www.press.uillinois.edu/journals/ethno.html

    Ethnomusicology is the official journal of the Society for Ethnomusicology. Articles reflect current theoretical work and empirical research in ethnomusicology and related fields. The journal is accessible to a diverse audience of musicians, musicologists, folklorists, popular culture scholars, and cultural anthropologists, and publishes a current bibliography, discography, and filmography, as well as book, record, and film reviews.

Music Perception
    ucpressjournals.com/journal.asp?jIssn=0730-7829

    Music Perception is a peer-reviewed journal that publishes empirical, theoretical, and methodological articles, as well as reviews. The range of disciplines covered in the journal include psychology, psychophysics, linguistics, neurology, neurophysiology, artificial intelligence, computer technology, physical and architectural acoustics, and music theory.

International Journal of Community Music
   www.intljcm.com/index.html

   The International Journal of Community Music is a peer-reviewed journal that publishes research articles, practical discussions, reviews, readers' notes, and special issues concerning all aspects of community music.

Studies in Musical Theatre
   www.intellectbooks.co.uk/journals.php?issn=17503159

   Studies in Musical Theatre is a peer-reviewed journal that publishes articles about live performance that uses vocal and instrumental music in conjunction with theatrical performance. Many aspects of the field are considered, including: opera, music theater or musical theater, actor musicianship, the training of performers for musical theater, the fusion of the languages of words and music, the use of music and song within "straight" theater, paralinguistics and the rhetorical expression of music in song, negotiating the art–entertainment divide in musical theater, and the academic study of musical theater. Book reviews are also published.

NOTE

1. For example, in Britain an urban musical genre called "British bhangra" has emerged and is now a popular style of music that is regularly played on radio and in dance clubs. This music combines elements of folk music from the Punjab people, located along the diverse and expansive borders of Pakistan and India, with black music genres and British pop music (Dudrah, 2002, p. 363). Specifically, British bhangra combines Punjabi lyrics, Indian drumbeats, the dhol, black musical genres, and British pop sounds (p. 363). Both the emergence of this hybrid genre of music and its acceptance into mainstream British music (and society) speak to larger issues pertaining to the arts, processes of cultural globalization, and identity negotiations among British South Asian audiences. According to Rajinder Dudrah (2002), this musical form speaks to a range of identity issues while affording listeners a space in which to create their own meanings. For example, this genre of music typically contains conservative lyrics with respect to gender and caste. In terms of gender, the industry that produces this music is male dominated, and thus heterosexual male fantasies about women as "objects of pleasure" abound, offering women limited roles in this medium (p. 376). In addition, caste-specific overtones permeate the music in highly gendered ways (p. 376). As British South Asian audiences listen to this music they may negotiate the meanings that emerge from it—for instance, although conservative lyrics are commonplace, the music is also fluid, flexible, and cross-cultural (p. 378). As evidenced by this example, musical hybrids are complex sites of identity negotiation and international exchange.

REFERENCES

Adorno, T. (1984). *Aesthetic theory* (C. Lendhardt, Trans; G. Adorno & R. Tiedemann, Eds.). London: Routledge.

Attali, J. (1985). *Noise: The political economy of music* (B. Massumi, Trans.). Minneapolis: University of Minnesota Press.

Anderson, W. M., Jr. (1974, Autumn). World music in American education. *Contributions to Music Education*, pp. 23–42.

Bhabha, H. (1993). Culture's in between. *Artform International, 32*(1), 167–171.

Bordo, S. (1993). *Unbearable weight: Feminism, Western culture, and the body*. Berkeley: University of California Press.

Bresler, L. (2005). What musicianship can teach educational research. *Music Education Research, 7*(2), 169–183.

Bresler, L., & Stake, R. E. (1992). Qualitative research methodology in music education. In R. Colwell (Ed.), *Handbook of music teaching and learning* (pp. 75–90). New York: Schirmer Books.

Butler, J. P. (1993). *Bodies that matter: On the discursive limits of sex*. London: Routledge.

Carrigan, N. (2003). Muscianship in the 21st century: Issues, trends and possibilities. In S. Leong (Ed.), *Thinking about Music: For a construction of meaning* (pp. 39–50). Sydney: Australian Music Centre.

Carter, W. L. (1973). Music in the black studies program. *The Black Perspective in Music, 1*(2), 147–150.

Casey, D. E. (1992). Descriptive research: Techniques and procedures. In R. Colwell (Ed.), *Handbook of music and teaching and learning* (pp. 115–123). New York: Schirmer Books.

Conquergood, D. (1985). Performing as a moral act: Ethical dimensions of the ethnography of performance. *Text and Performance Quarterly, 5*(2), 1–13.

Davis, C. S., & Ellis, C. (2008). Emergent methods in autoethnographic research: Autoethnographic narrative and the multiethnographic turn. In S. N. Hesse-Biber & P. Leavy (Eds.), *Handbook of emergent methods* (pp. 283–302). New York: Guilford Press.

Dudrah, R. K. (2002). British bhangra music and diasporic South Asian identity information. *European Journal of Cultural Studies, 5*(3), 363–383.

Elliot, D. J. (1989). Key concepts in multicultural music education. *International Journal of Music Education, 13*, 11–18.

Grossberg, M. (2005). Professor to present Korean narrative singing. *Columbus Dispatch*, p. 3.

Grosz, E. (1994). *Volatile bodies: Toward a corporeal feminism*. Bloomington: Indiana University Press.

Hesse-Biber, S. (1996). *Am I thin enough yet: The cult of thinness and the commercialization of identity*. New York: Oxford University Press.

Hesse-Biber, S. (2006). *The cult of thinness*. New York: Oxford University Press.

Hesse-Biber, S., & Leavy, P. (2006). *The practice of qualitative research*. Thousand Oaks, CA: Sage.

Holman Jones, S. H. (2002). Emotional space: Performing the resistive possibilities of torch singing. *Qualitative Inquiry, 8*(6), 738–759.

Jenoure, T. (2002). Sweeping the Temple: A performance collage. In C. Bagley & M. B. Cancienne (Eds.), *Dancing the data* (pp. 73–89). New York: Peter Lang.

Jordan, J. (1992). Handbook of research on music teaching and learning. In R. Caldwell (Ed.), *Multicultural music education in a pluralistic society* (pp. 735–748). New York: Schirmer Books.

Leavy, P., Gnong, A., & Sard-Ross, L. (2007). *Feminity, masculinity, and body image issues among college-age women: A multi-method interview study of mind–body dichotomy.* Manuscript under review.

Merleau-Ponty, M. (1962). *Phenomenology of perception* (C. Smith, Trans.). London: Routledge & Kegan Paul.

Morrison, A. (1992). The undisciplined muse: Music among the fields of knowledge. *Journal of Musicology, 10*(3), 405–415.

Pillow, W. S. (2001). Exposed methodology: The body as a deconstructive practice. *International Journal of Qualitative Studies in Education, 10*(3), 349–363.

Rhodes, W. (1963). Musicology and musical performance (comments on Hood, "Musical Significance"). *Ethnomusicology, 7*(3), 198–200.

Richardson, C. P., & Whitaker, N. L. (1992). Critical thinking and music education. In R. Colwell (Ed.), *Handbook of research on music teaching and learning* (pp. 546–560). New York: Schirmer Books.

Sprague, J., & Zimmerman, M. (1993). Overcoming dualisms: A feminist agenda for sociological method. In P. England (Ed.), *Theory on gender/feminism on theory.* New York: DeGruyter.

Spry, T. (2001). Performing autoethnography: An embodied methodological praxis. *Qualitative Inquiry, 7*(6), 706–732.

Stobin, M., & Titon, J. T. (1992). The music culture as a world of music. In J. T. Titon (Ed.), *Worlds of music: An introduction to the music of the world's peoples.* New York: Schirmer Books.

Stubley, E. V. (1995). The performer, the score, the work: Musical performance and transactional reading. *Journal of Aesthetic Education, 29*(3), 55–69.

Stubley, E. V. (1998). Being in the body, being in the sound: A tale of modulating identities and lost potential. *Journal of Aesthetic Education, 32*(4), 93–105.

Walker, R. (1992). Auditory–visual perception and musical behavior. In R. Colwell (Ed.), *Handbook of research on music teaching and learning* (pp. 344–359). New York: Schirmer Books.

Wolf, N. (1991). *The beauty myth.* New York: William Morrow.

The Role of Music
in an Arts-Based Qualitative Inquiry

Norma Daykin

Aesthetics as much as economics guides the interpretation of social life.
—SMITH (1997, p. 502)

This article explores the use of music as a potential research tool, drawing on research carried out by the author. Interest in arts-based research methods has grown in recent years as one consequence of an extended epistemology that recognizes different forms of knowledge (Reason, 1988, 1994). This explicitly draws on the evocative power of the arts in enhancing representation, generating new insights, and increasing understanding of phenomena (Norris, 1999, 2000, 2001). The move toward arts-based methodologies has also been linked with the postmodern trend toward the breaking down of disciplinary boundaries and the use of reflexive and situated accounts of research (Richardson, 1998). The claims made for arts-based methodologies relate to more than their decorative functions. For example, for Richardson, creative writing can act not just as a mopping-up exercise at the end of a project, but as a way of producing vital, situated texts and a "way of knowing" (p. 345). The creative process, she argues, enables us to discover new aspects of our topic and our relationship to it.

A review of arts-based methodologies provided by Joe Norris at a recent workshop[1] suggests that while creative writing, visual arts, film, photography, video, and theater-based performance are increasingly being used and evaluated in different research contexts, the use of arts that have neither a literary nor a visual basis is rare. In particular, music is infrequently used in research despite the increasing recognition of its evocative, educational, and healing powers in therapeutic and other settings (Boyce-Tillman, 2000; Bunt, 1994; Bunt & Hoskyns, 2002).

Music and Meaning

The infrequent use of music may reflect particular problems of interpretation, reflection upon which may be useful in the context of current debates about representation that, to some extent, underpin the case for arts-based research. Music certainly offers a powerful tool of expression, yet it may be difficult and even undesirable to pin down and exploit its meanings for research purposes.

Behind this debate lies the notion of aesthetic autonomy (Leppert, 1993; McClary, 2000; Williams, 2001), made particularly in relation to Western classical music, which may partially explain why music has received relatively little attention in the field of human inquiry. Since the 1980s, this notion has given way to a growing concern to explore the ways in which music generates meaning and how these meanings contribute to the reproduction of society and culture (Leppert, 1993, p. 16). The process of musical meanings has been linked with that of constructing and maintaining social hierarchies and identities (Leppert, 1993; McClary, 2000; Williams, 2001). There has also been increasing interest in the socioeconomic dimensions of taste and judgment and the notion of cultural capital in highlighting processes of status and advancement within particular fields (Bourdieu, 1984, 1993).

Yet the notion that the music "speaks for itself" has been a powerful one in music history. Hence, until relatively recently, issues of musical semantics have been treated with suspicion in mainstream music theory, which has focused inquiry on those questions "relating to the notes" (Leppert, 1993). As Williams (2001) suggests, while claims to aesthetic autonomy have increasingly given way to notions of music as socialized energies, the impact of these claims is still felt. Williams explores the influence of structuralism as a modernist musical project that reflects the scientific rationalism and the technocratic optimism of the immediate postwar period, seeking to locate quasi-automatic procedures in music and reduce subjectivity by limiting patterns of signification. Modernism is seen as valuing the internal unity within music at the expense of other elements, including external responses and affect. The influence of modernist ideas may to some extent account for the fact that music has not seemed accessible as a resource for research and inquiry processes. Yet the questions of meaning that arise from a consideration of reception and affect are clearly of importance to the development of an arts-based epistemology.

In McClary's (2000) view, claims of an aesthetic sphere that lies beyond the social serve represent a continuation of the elitism, essentialism, and conservativism of the Romantic period. While McClary's view is understandable in the light of the contemporary insights of sociomusicology, it is important to recognize that other, more democratic, impulses to protect musical values have influenced the debate. In this context, the potential of music to serve as an ideological tool in state nation-building projects (Shapiro, 2001) and other forms of social engineering (Frith, 2003) has been resisted. Many 20th-century composers have sought to distance themselves from disastrous associations between music and nationalism as well as cultural essentialism. The alignment of music with powerful forces has often been resisted, whether these relate to states or markets (Adorno, 1973).

It is in this postwar context that questions of music and meaning have been explored directly, both in text and sound. Composers such as Luciano Berio (1925–2003), influenced by the structural anthropology of Lévi-Strauss, have taken music to the limits of semantic meaning. A good example of this project is the second movement of Berio's *Sinfonia*, a composition for eight voices and orchestra. Written in 1968–1969, in its time this work was seen as an exemplary modernist manifesto (Whittall, 1999, p. 302). The second movement, "O King," is a tribute to the memory of Martin Luther King, whose name is stated at the end, only after its constituent sounds have been separated and handed back and forth between the voices.

While Berio recognized that the human voice always evokes connotative meanings, the signifying effects of vocal sounds are deliberately minimized in order to explore sonic meaning itself.[2] While the feeling of not understanding is important to the experience of listening, the music is undeniably evocative. Berio's music illustrates the complexity of the debate and the contingency of musical meaning, an important concern for those interested in arts-based research and one that extends to many nontextual representational forms. These concerns are explored in the rest of this article, which examines the limits and potential of music in arts-based inquiry, focusing on the three areas of representation, narrative, and empowerment.

Music and Representation

Early attempts by writers such as Cooke (1959) to associate particular melodic phrases or intervals with specific emotions seem naïve when we take into account the mediating effects on interpretation of culture, knowledge, repertoire, and experiences of listeners (Scott, 2000). For some, music can only make limited use of semiotics, as there is no systematic relationship between music and what it indicates. Hence music is a system of "signifiers without signifieds" (Tunstall, 1979, p. 44), a point that is well demonstrated in "O King." Yet as Williams (2001) suggests, music cannot represent events in the way of film or drama, but it can allude to them semiotically, leaving the listener to complete the rest of the event. Nevertheless, there cannot be simple and direct transfer of meaning through the chain of creator, performer, and listener, because "musical meaning emerges from a mix including the shreds of authorial intention, the voices inscribed in the text, and the subject positions of readers/listeners" (Williams, 2001, p. 61).

The problem of contingency may not relate to all texts, although musical "texts" pose particular problems. On the other hand, some postmodern researchers are seeking new means of engaging with contingency in order to overcome what are seen as the limitations of traditional accounts. For example, Marcus (1998) suggests that only in "messy texts" can we avoid the suggestion of linearity and coherence where these may not exist. Furthermore, such texts offer the ability to accommodate multiple identities and voices. Messy texts therefore engage with multiple meanings, conveying the whole without invoking totality. They resist the dominance of the researcher, recognizing that work is incomplete without readers' responses. In this light, music emerges as a useful textual form.

For some, arguments in favor of messy texts imply a relativist position that allows too much indiscriminate noise and abdicates the responsibility of interpretation. Yet qualitative data can be heterophonic: recognition of this in its interpretation does not necessarily lead to relativism. The problem for the researcher is that of portraying complex discussions in linear form. In music, such problems are managed through principles of orchestration, hence music is arguably able to encompass a greater degree of complexity than other representational forms. In music, voices can speak together without negating one another. A good illustrative example is the recent collaborative work by British jazz composer/saxophonist John Surman, with American drummer Jack DeJohnette, titled *Free and Equal* (2002). Here, woodwinds and brass represent different "voices" in an underlying text concerning troubled world politics. The work serves as a reminder of the principles of the United Nations 1948 *Universal Declaration of Human Rights*. Overall, the piece has a strong narrative structure. In the second movement, "Groundwork," voices enter in succession, each with its own motif or theme, and an increasingly complex texture is sustained. Each "voice" can be heard distinctly and none dominates or diminishes the others.

Of course, not everyone listening to this music will hear the underlying text. The music may be evocative for many reasons unrelated to the sources of its inspiration. It is apparent that there is a need to set the music up by presenting some kind of preamble if we are to use it as a useful means of exploration of any theme relating to human rights or the complexity of diversity. The music cannot speak for itself in any direct way. Hence, representation through music is only meaningful as part of a process in which actors are engaged. This, perhaps, limits the potential for musical works to serve as representational devices in their own right, if these are seen as an endpoint of research. In reality, good qualitative research continues to be reread and reinterpreted long after its initial publication.

If the value of music as representational device is limited, the discussion does point toward the benefits that might be gained from using music as an arts-based approach during those stages of any research process, including dissemination, in which importance is placed on working with others to generate, explore, and interpret diverse meanings and perspectives

Music and Narrative

While music may be incapable of generating direct semantic or semiotic meaning, McClary's (2000) work demonstrates the importance of narrative structure in giving meaning to musical forms. McClary highlights the ways in which music, through these structures, both reflects and helps to construct the social world. Here, there is an interesting parallel with qualitative methodologies of narrative analysis. Narrativization is seen as a universal process by which people make sense of experience, particularly in the light of disruptive events (Bury, 1982; Frank, 1995;

Riessman, 1993). Narrativization is not just an individual process: narrative analysts have highlighted the role of core narratives and plot forms as well as shared repertoires in shaping understandings of identity and the life course (Becker, 1997). As Frank (1995) suggests, stories have two sides: the personal and the social, and some narratives are privileged. Frank's work focuses on responses to health crises, and he notes the way in which Western societies favor restitution narratives, which in turn privilege the interests and perspectives of technocratic medicine. The narrative structure of restitution, in which the return to predictability is affirmed in the face of uncertainty, is contrasted with that of the quest narrative in which the acceptance of contingency is central. While restitution narratives reinforce the status quo, quest narratives seek to educate and empower, functioning both as memoir and manifesto.

The parallel between Frank's work and McClary's is strong, although the use of terminology is rather different. McClary (2000) focuses on the procedures of tonal music, which reflect 18th-century notions of subjectivity as well as values of rationality, individualism, and progress. Central to her analysis is the sonata form, which she characterizes as a quest narrative (her definition has much in common with Frank's notion of restitution). The music always begins and ends in the tonic key: no matter what unexplored territory is visited in between, the return to the known is guaranteed, thus original identity is affirmed. Within this form, musical procedures are seen as serving important social functions. Hence, important cadences both imply closure and stimulate desire for it, confirming audiences in their belief that rational effort results in the attaining of a goal:

> The self-motivated delay of gratification, which was necessary for the social world coming into being in the 18th century, worked on the basis of such habits of thought, and tonality teaches listeners how to live within such a world: how to project forward in time, how to wait patiently and confidently for the pay-off. (McClary, 2000, p. 67)

As Leppert (1993) has pointed out, the rituals of Western music cultures are closely linked with ideological forces. Hence, the concert-going etiquette of disciplined passivity and bodily control has been seen as mirroring macrocosmic processes of social order. What is presented as purely musical cannot be separated from the discourses that surround it: for example, the emphasis on foundation harmony as the basis of music is itself a reflection of Cartesian philosophy and the emergent natural science of 18th- and 19th-century Europe (Boyce-Tillman, 2000; Leppert, 1993).

McClary (2000) focuses on the conservative aspects of conventional procedures. These erase their ideological basis by seeming natural. The importance of McClary's work to the current debate is that it demonstrates the way in which narrative structures shape musical form, and the ways music itself can construct and constrain knowledge of the world. In relation to an arts-based epistemology, an important point is made by Williams (2001): narrative meanings need not take on conservative forms; music can also turn archetypes toward experiences they would normally exclude, thereby offering new insights and challenging so-called conventional wisdom.

Empowerment and Cultural Capital

While music has been examined as a social process with ideological foundations, music has also been seen as offering resources for challenging hegemonic ideologies, enabling cultural differentiation, giving voice to resistance, and challenging elite dominance over consumption and lifestyles (Ma, 2002). Smith (1997) explores the relationship between music and social empowerment through an exploration of the role of the brass band movement in industrial towns in northern England during the 1800s. In a climate where music as an art form was available only to a small segment of the population, Smith sees the brass band movement as allowing working-class people to appropriate the products of high culture for themselves. Furthermore, playing allowed individuals to achieve freedom of expression instrumentally in the context of a Victorian society where verbal expression of feelings and emotions was often not possible. While the higher social classes dismissed the artistic merits of brass band music, the music had a healing role in collective lives artificially split into labor and leisure (Smith, 1997, p. 514).

In the context of the arts-based research debate, Smith's (1997) work illustrates both the representational and the transformative power of music. As she suggests, "music has and constructs meaning: it can evoke a sense of space and of society that differs from, and is complementary to, that evoked by sight" (p. 524). Smith also draws parallels with Gilroy's (1993) analysis of the links between slavery and "black" musical forms, highlighting music's ability to communicate what cannot be spoken, articulating conditions of existence at the same time as establishing ownership of creative space and generating opportunities.

Music in Research: A Brief Example

These issues are being further explored in my own research in progress in the United Kingdom. The research is in two phases, with the second phase being a methodological development using music directly in the research process. It is this phase that this article addresses; however, in order to contextualize the discussion, brief details about the methodology and findings emerging from Phase One are presented.

The research began by exploring the impact of insecurity and ill health in the flexible world of music work. Within music work, finding acceptance within particular fields and in relation to particular aesthetic judgements is crucial to success. Such judgements are influenced by underlying ideas about the nature of creativity, which extend beyond the arts to include a range of spheres. Hence, the notion of creativity, both as a received idea and a personal discourse shaped by the musician/worker can be an important mediator of experience. The research used narrative analysis to explore notions of creativity as these were challenged and reworked in response to disruptions such as ill health. Thirteen freelance musicians, identified through networks and through an article in a professional journal, were interviewed. Full details of this research are available elsewhere (Daykin, in press); only a brief overview is provided here to aid the discussion.

Narrative analysts suggest that narrativisation is itself a response to threats to identity that are encountered when one's own life events mean that one cannot fulfill an expected life course (Becker, 1997; Frank, 1995). People tell stories to make sense of their experiences. While these may be personal stories, they often have broader cultural significance, relating to wider themes such as medicalization and power (Frank, 1995). Hence, core narratives can emerge that link personal storytelling with broader cultural processes (Bury, 1982). In the current research, narrative reworkings were often reworkings of creativity discourse. Conventional notions of creativity seem to draw on assumptions of creativity as an innate characteristic, a "gift" enjoyed by the privileged few. Narrative structures linked with this notion portray the artist, usually male, as hedonistic, encountering great risks and enduring great suffering, isolated from society (Boyce-Tillman, 2000). These core narratives exercise a powerful influence on the individual's sense of creative identity and entitlement, both of which can be seriously challenged, not just by illness but by having the "wrong" gender, sexual, or ethnic identity as well as the chronic strains of insecure and relatively unregulated work. Individuals seeking to engage in such work must define themselves in relation to conventional notions of creativity within their particular field, and attempting to live up to perceived norms is sometimes seen as a source of ill-being if not ill health and injury (Daykin, in press).

Phase One of my research focused on the key metaphors that emerged from narrative reworkings of creative identity. These metaphors allowed individuals to continue to make claim to creativity, and therefore to continue to participate in work, while at the same time acknowledging the contingencies of vulnerability and risk. Here three examples are offered. First, the metaphor of pacing was often used to counter the notion that creative activity is driven, obsessive and disembodied. Second, the notion of connection often provided a key narrative resource, in contrast with ideas of aggressive competition and individualism that were seen as characterizing some forms of music work. Finally, some accounts drew explicitly on the notion of service: focusing on the needs of others (readers, listeners, students, communities) was seen as counterbalancing particular concerns, such as performance anxiety. These stories are more than individuals' attempts to make sense of crises and chronic strains, they represent a cultural critique of dominant notions of creativity at work that serve to reward some identities and diminish others.

Phase Two of the research is a methodological development that arose from the process of interpretation of the data. As the stories unfolded, it became clear that each existed in a particular sound world. For example, as people described the changes in their instrumental technique or approach to performance that had sometimes been forced by difficult circumstances, they also engaged in an aesthetic reevaluation of particular forms of music as well as new ways of playing or writing. Appreciation of these sound worlds seems an important dimension of listening to these particular stories.

Hence, Phase Two of the research focuses explicitly on these sound worlds, exploring their impact both as representational devices and as a means of generating new insights. Each participant is invited to offer particular music that is meaningful to them in the context of the themes emerging from the research interview. The interview process then extends to discuss these meanings, and the process continues as the research is disseminated and each new audience considers the research themes, assisted partly through the medium of sound.

As well as the methodological issues raised by the research, ethical issues that may be similar to those in other arts-based methodologies have arisen. One of these is the tension between the conventional principle of anonymity in research and the ethical requirement that creative work be credited. Many of the contributions offered by participants are original works. In each case, the issue of informed consent needs to be examined both from the perspective of arts and research. No one is required to surrender anonymity, but often people prefer their work and their thinking on these issues to be known.

To illustrate the discussion, I focus an example of a work by a British composer, Tony Osborne, who has taken part in the research and who has agreed to be identified. Part of the interview and subsequent conversations with Tony have been about the relationship between music and healing on a personal level and whether this meaning is sustained when music is received by others. As Osborne says:

> For me composing is always a healing process one way or another. It can sometimes be a statement of something deep inside me—or inside the recipient, or some other person or issue. In this way, perhaps it is a partial "exorcism" of a kind.
>
> I always like it if the spirit/life-force, or emotional atmosphere of a piece comes through—for performers and listeners, but I don't regard it as a failure if it doesn't, as each is an individual. I equally like it if it is received in a different way, or indeed if it just serves as superficial reaction—whatever it is, or is just wallpaper to escape into. I like others to form their own pictures and impressions—or none!

One of the works in question is from the first movement of *Melodic Portraits,* a double-bass concerto dedicated to John Walton.[3] It was written as part of the process of healing that occurred after the death of Walton, one of Osborne's former teachers. It is strongly evocative and seeks to reflect the composer's view of Walton's inner spirit. Rather than being purely representational, however, an important issue emerged from the discussion: that new meanings can be generated from music:

> It can also be a reverse process and instill in me something that I did not feel—a new feeling, a new perspective of something or someone, a new discovery. ... It's difficult to be too specific, but I believe I've sensed any or all of these things at some time or other.

Conclusion

Ultimately, the meanings generated by music in any research process are specific and contextual. Yet the same can be said of many texts whose meaningfulness is often taken for granted in qualitative research. As has been argued here, some art forms, and specifically music, cannot speak for themselves. In this instance, understanding particular stories is made more complete by consideration of the sound worlds that they inhabit and produce. Hence, there is evidence that the use of music in particular forms of research may be useful, not just in enhancing representation but in considering new elements and dimensions of data. Furthermore, this paper has identified the potentially transformative power of music-making in the context of cultural notions of creativity that both enhance and diminish particular identities and contributions. Hence, arts-based research processes may be particularly beneficial in action-oriented research processes. In conclusion, it is suggested that music and music-making can offer useful resources for inquiry, as well as highlight some important problems of contingency that are of broader significance in the context of new insights claimed for arts-based research.

Notes

1. Preconference workshop held in conjunction with the Fifth Advances in Qualitative Methods Conference, January 29, 2004, in Edmonton, Alberta, Canada.
2. I am grateful to Tim Raymond, head of composition at Royal Welsh College of Music and Drama, for this observation.
3. For further information about this work, please contact the author at *norma.daykin@uwe.ac.uk*.

References

Adorno, T. (1973). *Philosophy of modern music*. London: Sheen and Ward.

Becker, G. (1997). *Disrupted lives: How people create meaning in a chaotic world*. London: University of California Press.

Berio, L. (1969). *Sinfonia* [Pierre Boulez, French National Orchestra]. On *Sinfonia, Eindrücke* [CD]. Paris: Erato. (Recorded April 1984).

Bourdieu, P. (1984). *Distinction: A social critique of the judgment of taste*. Cambridge, MA: Harvard University Press.

Boyce-Tillman, J. (2000). *Constructing musical healing: The wounds that sing*. London: Kingsley.

Bunt, L. (1994). *Music therapy: An art beyond words*. London: Routledge.

Bunt, L., & Hoskyns, S. (Eds.). (2002). *The handboook of music therapy*. London: Brunner-Routledge.

Bury, M. (1982). Chronic illness as biographical disruption. *Sociology of Health and Illness, 4*(2), 167–182.

Cooke, D. (1959). *The language of music*. Oxford, UK: Oxford University Press.

Daykin, N. (in press). Disruption, dissonance and embodiment, creativity, health and risk in music narratives. *Health*.

Frank, A. W. (1995). *The wounded storyteller: Body, illness and ethics*. London: University of Chicago Press.

Frith, S. (2003). Music and everyday life. In M. Clayton, T. Herbert, & R. Middleton (Eds.), *The cultural study of music: A critical introduction* (pp. 92–101). London: Routledge.

Gilroy, P. (1993) *The black Atlantic: Modernity and double consciousness.* Cambridge, MA: Harvard University Press.

Leppert, R. (1993). *The sight of sound: Music, representation, and the history of the body.* Berkeley: University of California Press.

Ma, E. (2002). Emotional energy and subcultural politics: Alternative bands in post-1997 Hong Kong. *Inter-Asia Cultural Studies, 3*(2), 187–200.

Marcus, G. E. (1998). What comes (just) after "Post"¿: The case of ethnography. In N. K. Denzin & Y. S. Lincoln (Eds.), *The landscape of qualitative research: Theories and issues* (pp. 383–406). London: Sage.

McClary, S. (2000). *Conventional wisdom: The content of musical form.* Berkeley: University of California Press.

Norris, J. (1999). Creative drama as adults work. In B. J. Wagner (Ed.), *Building moral communities through educational drama* (pp. 217–237). Stamford, CT: Ablex.

Norris, J. (2000). Drama as research: Realizing the potential of drama in education as a research methodology. *Youth Theatre Journal, 14,* 40–51.

Norris, J. (2001). Using drama in teaching language arts. In G. Tompkins, M. Pollard, R. Bright, & P. Winsor (Eds.), *Language arts: Content and teaching strategies* (2nd ed., pp. 284–321). Toronto: Prentice-Hall.

Reason, P. (1988). *Human inquiry in action: Developments in new paradigm research.* London: Sage.

Reason, P. (Ed.). (1994). *Participation in human inquiry.* London: Sage.

Richardson, L. (1998). Writing: A method of inquiry. In N. K. Denzin & Y. S. Lincoln (Eds.), *Collecting and interpreting qualitative materials* (pp. 345–371). London: Sage.

Riessman, C. K. (1993). *Narrative analysis.* London: Sage.

Scott, D. B. (2000). Music and language: Introduction. In D. B. Scott (Ed.), *Music, culture, and society: A reader* (pp. 21–27). Oxford, UK: Oxford University Press.

Shapiro, M. J. (2001). Images and narratives in world politics. *Millennium, 30*(3), 583–602.

Smith, S. J. (1997). Beyond geography's visible worlds: A cultural politics of music. *Progress in Human Geography, 21*(4), 502–529.

Surman, J. (2002). Groundwork. On *Free and Equal* [CD]. Munich: ECM.

Tunstall, P. (1979). Structuralism and musicology: An overview. *Current Musicology, 27,* 61–63.

Whittall, A. (1999). *Musical composition in the twentieth century.* Oxford, UK: Oxford University Press.

Williams, A. (2001). *Constructing musicology.* Ashgate, UK: Aldershot.

CHAPTER 5

Performance Studies

> The performance text is the single, most powerful way for ethnography
> to recover yet interrogate the meanings of lived experience.
> —Norman K. Denzin (1997, pp. 94–95)

Performance exists in the moment and it is immediate. A performance event is both temporal and ephemeral in that an artifact such as a video recording may remain, but not the event itself (Saldaña, 1999). Perhaps more than anything else, performance-based methods can bring research findings to life, adding dimensionality, and exposing that which is otherwise impossible to authentically (re)present. Saldaña writes:

> … theatre is one of the artistic media through which fictionalized and non-fictionalized social life—the human condition—can be portrayed symbolically and aesthetically for spectator engagement and reflection. (2005, p. 10)

Congruent with the move toward public sociology, performances are accessible to diverse audiences and constitute an exchange or transfer between the audience and performer(s) (and the script). Moreover, the "exchange" may involve a complex negotiation of meanings. This interaction between the performer and audience also varies depending on the environment and mood (Langellier & Peterson, 2006).

In social research, performance can serve many research purposes, including consciousness-raising, empowerment, emancipation, political agendas, discovery, exploration, and education. Although often considered a representational form, performance can be used as an entire research method, serving as a means of data collection and analysis as well as a (re)presentation form. Moreover, theories of performance are often entangled with methodological practices. Performance is therefore an investigation *and* a representation (Worthen, 1998). In addition, data collected via more traditional qualitative research methods, such as ethnography and interview, can be translated into performance texts in many different ways.

The performance genre has affected the qualitative paradigm in ways that indicate performance extends beyond a method or representational form and offers a new way of thinking about and conducting social research. In this regard, Gray (2003) argues that performance challenges and disrupts conventional ways of knowing (p. 254). Oikarinen-Jabai (2003) suggests that a performance-based methodology allows researchers to transgress borders with their research participants and serves as a means for locating empowering spaces, exposing contradictions, and building empathy (p. 578). Writing about her experience with this kind of methodology, Oikarinen-Jabai concludes, "A performative approach helps me to find, experience, and express the desire, passion, ambivalence, powerlessness, uncertainty, shame, love, fear, and other emotions that are hidden in our relationships and our cultural discourses" (p. 578).

The use of performance as a research method has exploded over the last three decades, making performance perhaps the most widely used method in this book. There are many variations on how performance serves qualitative methodology as well as many catalysts for this major trend in research practice; therefore, this chapter reviews a selection of these practices.

For scholars working within the theater arts, the recent surge in social researchers drawing on the power of performance is not surprising. There is an affinity between the work of playwriting and performing and the craft of qualitative research. Johnny Saldaña (1999) proposes that there is a similarity between the goal of qualitative researchers and playwrights, both of whom try "to create a unique, engaging, and insightful text about the human condition" (p. 60). He further asserts that theatre practitioners have the following foundational qualitative research skills:

1. Enhanced sensory awareness and observation skills, enabling an attuned sensitivity to fieldwork environments
2. The ability to analyze characters and dramatic texts, which transfers to analyzing interview transcripts and fieldnotes for participant actions and relationships

3. The ability to infer objectives and subtext in participants' verbal and nonverbal actions, which enriches social insight

4. Scenographic literacy, which heightens the visual analysis of field-work settings, space, artifacts, participant dress, etc.

5. The ability to think conceptually, symbolically, and metaphorically—essentials for qualitative data analysis

6. An aptitude for storytelling, in its broadest sense, which transfers to the writing of engaging narrative research reports (p. 68)

Similarly, Joe Norris (2000) argues that practitioners of drama education have tremendous experience with drama as a *meaning-making method* as well as a (re)presentational form. For example, Norris explains that in drama classrooms students routinely test hypotheses "through the magic of what if" (p. 41). Citing Berry and Reinbold (1985), Norris argues that practices in educational drama can be considered a research methodology and refers to *collective creation,* which is a play that is created by the entire cast as a series of vignettes. This technique, referred to as "play building" by Tarlington and Michaels (1995), draws on the same techniques qualitative researchers use in their meaning-making processes. Norris writes, "Much of what we do in process drama helps us to re-look at content to draw insights and make new meanings; this act can be considered a research tool" (p. 44).

The connection between theater arts and qualitative research has been discovered and explored as a result of a series of simultaneous developments within academic scholarship. The move toward performance, or what Victor Turner (1974) deems a "performance paradigm," is linked to developments in embodiment research and the mind–body connection (elaborated elsewhere in this book), postmodern theoretical advancements (in this regard Denzin, 1997, refers to the "sublime" postmodern performance text), the larger academic move to interdisciplinary and multidisciplinary scholarship, as well as the cumulative impact of researchers expanding and refining the qualitative paradigm in accord with new theoretical, epistemological, and methodological innovations (in particular, researchers looking for ways to access subjugated voices).

McLeod (1988) argues against the idea that there are only two ways of making meaning (i.e., qualitative and quantitative) and advances a theory of five ways of making meaning (i.e., word, number, image, gesture, and sound), which Norris (2000) proposes are all integrated in drama. Performance methods are congruent with holistic views of the research process.

Performance studies merge advances in embodiment research, the move to integrate the mind and body in social research, and the move to cross or blur disciplinary boundaries in an attempt to access subjugated perspectives. As in lived experience, there is no separation between the mind and body in the context of performance. Moreover, the performers and audience members are embodied actors, marked by gendered, raced, sexed, and classed discursive practices.

Langellier and Peterson (2006) suggest that performance studies cross boundaries and expose "the cracks of disciplinary boundaries" (p. 153). Moreover, the "I" and the "you" may find themselves in symbiosis in the performance of personal narratives (p. 156). In this regard, Langellier and Peterson write, "Performing personal narrative reclaims and proclaims both body and voice: the personal gives a body to narrative, and narrative gives voice to experience" (p. 156). Moreover, performance serves as a method for exposing what is otherwise impossible to reveal. This potential results from the three main qualities of performance that Langellier and Peterson define as framed, reflexive, and emergent. They write:

> First a breakthrough performance is framed, that is, marked off from surrounding discourse and keyed by performance conventions of particular speech communities. The performance frame strikes a contract of mutual risk taking and responsibility between performer and audience to "take this communication in a special way": as a storytelling event. Second, performance is reflexive because the performer is audience to her or his own experience and turns back to signify this lived work with and for an audience. The storyteller narrates turning points in returning to experience; performance is a doing and a redoing that allows scrutiny of experience; self, and world. ... Third performance has the potential of emergence, that is, in redoing something one may do it differently. (p. 155)

Similarly, W. B. Worthen (1998), noting the methodological strengths of performances, explains that they can be unmade and remade (p. 1101).

Although very recent epistemological, theoretical, and methodological developments have promoted the expansion of the performance paradigm, sociologists have long recognized that performance is an inseparable component of social life. In this regard, Erving Goffman (1959) coined the term "dramaturgy" to denote the presentation of self that people engage in during their daily lives. Building on the famous idea that "all the world's a stage and we are but the actors on it," Goffman posited that in social life there is a "front stage" and "backstage." The front stage is what others see (in theater, this would be the actual performance); and the backstage is all of the behind-the-scenes stuff of life that others do not see (in theater, this would be the playwriting, the rehearsals, hair and makeup, etc.). Under this theoretical framework, all of life involves performance, including what Goffman termed "face-saving" strategies. In a similar vein, Worthen (1998) notes that social life is full of performances such as street performances, identity performances, and everyday life as drama.

Postmodern scholarship has also contributed to our understanding of the complexity of performance in social life. For example, Judith Butler (1993) theorizes about the performance of gender by discursively constituted and constituting subjects. Performance can also be a space where identity categories are renegotiated, struggled over, and challenged. Connected to postmodern theory, scholarship on hybridity has also influenced our understanding of performance and identity work.

Homi Bhabha (1993) writes about the hybrid "third space" (created when two cultural forms merge) that cannot be understood by traditional conceptual frameworks. Influenced by his work, Helena Oikarinen-Jabai (2003) writes about the performances of the Gambian women she researched and how these performances served to challenge discursively constituted identities.

> The performances of Gambian women made me admire their ability to challenge their cultural and gendered identities and to use different and traditional and imported genres in criticizing and questioning cultural conventions and hierarchies. They connect art to their everyday experience. (p. 576)

The anthropological study of performance, as well as concepts of drama in everyday life, influence performance-based methodological practices, although they themselves are not the subject of this chapter.

Drama as a Means of Personal Growth, Consciousness-Raising, and Subversion

Many of the epistemological and theoretical positions that in recent decades have changed the face of the qualitative paradigm also promote an exchange between researcher and researched that is not only more collaborative and egalitarian but also actively beneficial to the research participants. In this context, the consciousness-raising and empowering potential of drama has become an instigator for performance-based methodological development. In a general sense, drama is a form of communication that can foster personal growth (Warren, 1993). As drama utilizes imagination, it can assist people in examining how their life is and how they would like it to be (Warren, 1993). Moreover, in addition to imagination drama cultivates flexibility, expression, and even social skills (Warren, 1993).

Norman K. Denzin (2006) writes about the pedagogical dimensions of performance when it is employed as a critical pedagogy, including (1) as a form of instruction that helps people to think critically, historically, and sociologically; (2) as a means of exposing the pedagogies of oppression; and (3) as a means of contributing to an ethical self-consciousness that will help shape a critical race awareness (p. 332). In addition, *performance pedagogy* fosters the "sociological imagination," allowing participants to reveal and explore the link between historical processes and their individual biographies (p. 332). Denzin asserts that promoting this kind of critical self-reflection and consciousness-raising is a political act with the potential to challenge normalized viewpoints. In this regard, he writes that through performance pedagogy "a critical consciousness is invoked" (p. 330). Going even further with respect to the possibilities for empowerment and subversion, Denzin writes: "Critical Pedagogical Theatre can empower persons to be subversive, while making their submission to oppression disappear" (p. 331). Here an excellent empirical example comes from Kristin Bervig Valentine's (2006) research on incarcerated women and performance.

Valentine (2006) suggests that creating a performance space for women in prison allows the women an otherwise impossible outlet for expression. For example, performance is the only space in which a statement such as "fuck the guards" is permissible (p. 315). She further proposes that this kind of programming reduces recidivism (p. 313). Valentine writes:

> My hypothesis is that mind-liberating activities generated by performance and creative writing programs ... increase effective communication skills that help women avoid actions harmful to themselves and others. By acquiring these skills they increase their abilities to avoid reincarceration when they are released from prison, thereby benefiting themselves, their families, and their communities. (p. 321)

In these ways and others, drama can be a vehicle for self-expression in ways tied to consciousness-raising, self-reflection, and subversion.

Another example comes from Claudio Moreira's (2005) research in which he explores dramatic performance as a method for revealing the experiences of the oppressed class in Brazil, and more specifically how the dominant class determines what people learn (a process that contributes to a cycle of oppression). Moreira's paper is constructed as a performative text in which each voice is a person sitting in the audience, so that when they stand up to speak they are a part of the audience. Together the voices tell the story of a young boy who lives in a poor neighborhood in Brazil. He learns from the other boys the sexist and racist idea that young black girls are "made for sex." The audience follows his thoughts as he gathers with other boys to conspire to rape black girls. Interwoven with this narrative of horror are messages about "dominant narratives" and how they are constructed by media writers and others with the power to disseminate ideologies that perpetuate a cycle of ignorance and oppression in which the oppressed victimize one another while they are simultaneously deterred from examining the source of their "commonsense" ideas. Moreira writes:

> This "knowledge" has been (in)formed and shaped in the same way that the images of friends of mine and myself were formed in childhood, by stories, conversations about what the people had experienced, by documentaries and news, magazines and newspapers. This knowledge is, in large part, the result of the dominant hegemonic narratives that are not only available to all but also make those beliefs seem natural and unchangeable. (p. 3)

This research illustrates another forum in which a dramatic structure can facilitate critical reflection, awareness, and the expression of subjugated voices.

Drama as a Research Activity: Drama as Data Collection, Analysis, and Representation

As noted earlier, Joe Norris (2000) posits that drama can serve as a complete research activity, with the potential to serve as a method of data collection, analysis, and (re)presentation (p. 45). Drawing on Donmoyer and Yennie-Donmoyer (1995) he articulates the intimate relationship between form and content in performance-based research and then notes that this intimacy is paralleled in the relationship between analysis and representation. He explains that in Readers' Theatre the way data are structured constitutes a form of analysis. For example, the placement of quotes is an *analytic act*. Readers' Theatre and "staged readings" have become popular presentation styles at conferences (Norris, 2000, p. 43).

Norris likens the dramatic process to the qualitative practice of focus groups. Similar to a focus group, a cast gathers to examine a particular topic or question; however, differing from the "moderator" role researchers adopt in focus groups, within the context of a dramatic "collective creation" there is no division between the researcher and participants. The cast (referred to as the informants in traditional qualitative research) provide the initial data, out of which a performance emerges via a drama-based process of analysis and dissemination. Writing of his experience with improvisation as a meaning-making activity Norris proclaims,

> In the improvisation the researchers/actors articulated what they knew (data collection); framed it in the improvisation (analysis); and presented it to others (dissemination). Consequently, improvisation, even in its rudimentary form, is a research act. (2000, p. 44)

Readers' Theatre and related collaborative drama-based methods can utilize data collected from traditional qualitative methods.

For example, Finley (1998) presented a Readers' Theatre piece based on interviews with homeless people in New Orleans. Out of these interviews Finley created composite characters as "types" of youth identified in the data. The dramatic presentation of the data, in which each character spoke in the first person, allowed Finley to get at some of the authentic experience in a way that would not have been possible with traditional representational forms. When working with these kinds of dramatic methods, the data do not need to be collected in a conventional way. Data can also come from public sources.

Norris has been commissioned by outside agencies to create performance pieces and workshops on many subjects. He has collaborated to create dramatic pieces exploring a diverse range of topics, including violence in schools, inclusion/exclusion, prejudice, sexuality, body image, addiction, equality/respect in the workplace, risk-taking, and student teaching. He advocates a "spiral process" of play-building in which all of the phases inform each other and the entire process has a dramatic structure (2000, pp. 46–48). As a part of this methodology he has created a record keeping system that he likens to "coding." Conceptualizing "record keeping" or "coding" as an "emergent process," he advocates using a series of files in which cast members place note cards with their thoughts, ideas, impressions, and so forth throughout the process. Some of the files he uses are: "To Be Filed," "Themes/Issues," "Metaphors," "Scene Ideas," "Rehearsed Scenes," "Quickies" (short scenes and phrases), "Keepers," "Props/Costumes/Music Needs," "External

Research Data," and "Potential Titles" (p. 47). In this way, the analytic and writing process has reflexivity built into it (p. 46). Ultimately, as the performance approaches Norris notes a shift occurs from collection to compilation—a process guided by the question "What do we want this play to be about?" (p. 47). Similarly, one could develop data directly from a literature review. In this kind of project, the literature review takes center stage in the knowledge-building process.

The remainder of this chapter reviews some of the major methodological practices in performance studies. Various performance methods as well as strategies for building a performance-based research design are addressed, as are issues of validity, authenticity, and ethics.

Script and Performance-Based Research Methods

Performances are distinct from performance scripts or texts. In the following section I review some of the ways in which performance scripts are constructed, primarily with the intent of being "performed"; however, it should be noted that performance scripts can be created without a performance happening. In other words, the script format can be used solely as a writing vehicle. This is different from wholly performance-based research, which stems from enactment.

Ethnographic Performance Texts

Ethnographic performance texts can be understood as textual representations of research data. This form of representation mirrors the form of playwriting. In other words, these performance texts are data-informed *scripts*. The resulting script may be the final stage of a research project; however, more often the script is *performed*. When an ethnographic performance text is performed, it could be for a multitude of purposes, including as the final representational stage, as a medium for garnering additional data, or as an analytical phase for the purpose of refining the script.

Yvonna S. Lincoln (2004) assembled a performance text with several colleagues to create a discourse about how people can get past silences that flow from the events of September 11th and the dominant American response to it. The piece is titled "Performing 9/11: Teaching in a Terrorized World," and it explores many issues. For example, the scholars explore the issue of teaching social subjects in a context in which dissent is viewed as unpatriotic. In essence, the piece explores how to get past the silence (to this end, a Greek chorus serves to disrupt silence in the script, showing how metaphor can serve meaning-making). The following is an excerpt from the performance text written by Norman K. Denzin:

> In the weeks after 9/11/01 everywhere I looked, I saw flags of every type, size, and shape: flag pens, flag mousepads, flag stickers, flags on poles that waved in the wind, flags on coffee cups, flags on radio antennas, big, little, and medium-sized flags. Flags so big they covered football fields. Songs about flags became popular, songs with lines like "Red, White, and Blue, these colors don't run."
>
> Last Spring a woman in Urbana, Illinois, made up a questionnaire and asked storekeepers why they had flags in their windows. "I was just curious," she replied, when asked why she had done this. Store owners reacted in anger and accused her of being a troublemaker. People called the local talk radio station and wrote letters to the editor of our local paper. They said she was being unpatriotic. (quoted in Lincoln, 2004, p. 142)

As you can see, in this example the performance text method was used as a method of incorporating different voices into a discourse, challenging a space of silence, exploring the relationship between the personal and political, accessing the experiences of some people within a particular social climate, and revealing the perspective of those Americans targeted as unpatriotic after September 11th as a result of exhibiting their political dissent. In short, the performance text is a method of getting at and illuminating a range of issues that are not accessible via traditional research methodologies.

Ethnodrama, Ethnotheater, and Performance Ethnography

Ethnodrama and ethnotheater are perhaps the most widely used performance-based methods. *Ethnodrama* refers to the writing up of research findings in dramatic or script form and may or may not be performed. Saldaña writes:

> An ethno*drama*, the written script, consists of dramatized, significant selections of narrative collected through interviews, participant observation field notes, journal entries, and/or print and media artifacts such as diaries, television broadcasts, newspaper articles, and court proceedings ... this is dramatizing the data. (2005, p. 2)

Ethnotheater is a performance-based method, constituted by a dramatic event (such as the live performance of an ethnodrama). "Ethnotheater" and "performance ethnography" are terms often used interchangeably, and speak to a particular subset of practices within performance studies. This group of performance-based methods relies on using qualitative data garnered from ethnography, interviews, public documents, and other traditional qualitative research methods and then analyzing, interpreting, and representing the data via a dramatic script. Saldaña (2005) writes the following:

> Ethno*theatre* employs the traditional craft and artistic techniques of theatre production to mount for an audience a live performance event of research participants' experiences and/or the researcher's interpretation of data. (p. 1)

The move by some qualitative researchers toward ethnodrama results from the ability of dramatic performance to get at and present rich, textured, descriptive, situated, contextual experiences and multiple meanings from the perspectives of those studied in the field. In other words, there is an affinity between ethnodramatic performance and the general principles of ethnography that guide many qualitative researchers. Moreover, the theater arts allow qualitative researchers to explore the dimensionality, tonality, and multisensory experiences that occur within the field in ways not enabled by traditional textual representation. This allows the audience deeper access to the raw data, in a manner of speaking.

- How can a researcher write an ethnodrama?
- What strategies are available for the analysis and interpretation of traditional qualitative data garnered through ethnography, interviews, and the like, with the goal of constructing an ethnodramatic script for performance? What coding issues arise? What ethical issues?
- What components of typical theater arts playwriting must a qualitative researcher consider when writing an ethnodrama? How is the process similar or dissimilar to solely artistic playwriting?
- What is the process by which research participants are transformed into characters? How does dialogue or monologue emerge?
- What are the plotting, story-lining, and structural components that frame the narrative and communicate meaning?
- What visual elements enter the meaning-making process?

Johnny Saldaña (1998, 1999, 2003, 2005) has written extensively about the practice of ethnodrama. As with any research project, he proposes that ethnodrama be employed when it serves the goals of a particular project and he suggests that researchers ask themselves how the story they seek to tell can be "validly, vividly, and persuasively told" (1999,

p. 61). Saldaña focuses primarily on the process by which researchers can analyze, interpret, and represent their data as an ethnographic performance.

Although all research involves a reduction process by which raw data are sorted through and condensed, made particularly salient in qualitative research, Saldaña suggests that this process occurs in a particular context in performance studies where the researcher aims to reduce the data to "the juicy stuff" in order to achieve dramatic impact (1999, p. 61). The desire to retain the "juicy stuff" is not without its own set of issues. Saldaña (1998) discovered a host of ethical considerations linked to this aspect of producing a performance text. During a study about an adolescent aspiring actor named "Barry," Saldaña encountered several ethical dilemmas when Barry and his parents experienced some unanticipated conflicts. Casting choices came into question, and some of the information revealed during private in-depth interviews constituted "the juicy stuff," but its use may have jeopardized the privacy of the participants. These issues notwithstanding, how does one construct an ethnodrama?

Reviewing the different components of a script, Saldaña (1999) provides a step-by-step list of issues researchers confront as they attempt to create ethnographic performance texts. As with all qualitative research, the coding procedure implemented is vital to the construction of the text, and this is enhanced in performance texts because analysis and representation occur fluidly. Saldaña advocates *in vivo coding*, where the participants' own words are used as coding labels during the analytic process because such categories may later assist the researcher as he or she determines which passages should be used for dialogue and monologues. Grounded theory methods of analysis and other inductive approaches can also accomplish this end. *Grounded theory* involves an inductive coding process in which data are analyzed, typically line-by-line, and code categories emerge directly out of the data (see Charmaz, 2008, for a discussion of emergent grounded theory practices). The categories and themes that emerge during this process may eventually become scenes in the play (Saldaña, 1999, p. 61). There are several major components of the play that must be worked through: characters, dialogue/monologues, plotting, structures, scenography, and costuming.

In ethnographic and interview research the participants are the locus of meaning and are central to the research process. Therefore, although the different components of plays may be constructed in any number of arrangements, I begin with a review of character development.

Saldaña (1999, 2003) proposes that the number of research participants whose stories stand out during a review of the data become the number of characters in the script. Characters in the script can be constructed as composites so that the themes that emerged during data collection—which in interviews, for example, may have come forth in multiple interviews—can be used to create character "types." This is the method Finley (1998) employed in her Readers' Theatre about homeless youth in New Orleans. The number of characters and their relation to one another affect the plot and structure of the play as well. For example, the play may unfold from the perspective of a central character (the protagonist), two characters in conflict (protagonist and antagonist), two flawed characters who guide each other to greater understanding, multiple characters in vignettes, or other standard formats (Saldaña, 1999).

Although researchers who create dramatic scripts have a range of dramatic/artistic considerations, revealing "truth" with respect to the research participants also compels the script construction. In this regard, Saldaña (1999, p. 62) provides guidelines for how researchers can create three-dimensional portrayals.

1. from interviews: what the participant reveals about his or her perceptions;

2. from fieldnotes, journal entries, or memoranda: what the researcher observes, infers, and interprets from the participant in action;

3. from observations or interviews with other participants connected to the primary case study: perspectives about the primary participant; and

4. from the research literature: what other scholars and theorists offer about the phenomena under study.

Directly linked to characterization is the issue of dialogue and monologue. In ethnodrama the dialogue or monologue may be extracted directly from the raw data (e.g., an excerpt from an interview transcript), or the text may be constructed by the researcher during the interpretive process. Saldaña posits that dialogue can reveal how characters react to one another (which may particularly appeal to researchers working from a symbolic interactionist framework), and that monologues, when done well, can offer social insight (which may include the researcher's voice or voices from the literature review or theory) and can also foster an emotional response from the audience (this connection being vital to performance-based methods) (Saldaña, 1999, pp. 63–66). The relationship between the characters and their dialogue is dialectical. For example, when composite characters are created out of multiple participants' stories the researcher then considers this when he or she writes the dialogue. Saldaña (1999, p. 64) offers the following guidelines:

> Participant voices come from two or more individual interviews can be interwoven to:
>
> 1. offer triangulation through their supporting statements;
> 2. highlight disconfirming evidence from their contrast and juxtaposition; and/or
> 3. exhibit collective story creation through the multiplicity of perspectives.

In addition, the researcher must consider his or her own role within the script. This is a concern for all qualitative researchers, made explicit in the case of performance texts. For example, there is a great body of literature about "sharing authority" in the research process, particularly with respect to methodologies that rely on the co-construction of knowledge that occurs as researchers and participants collaborate (see Frisch, 1990). Feminist researchers, particularly those working in the tradition of oral history and ethnography, have been at the forefront of discussions about hierarchy, collaboration, authority, disclosure, voice, and reflexivity in the knowledge-building process. In ethnodrama the place of the researcher within the process, an epistemological decision, becomes explicit as the researcher must decide how to write him- or herself into the script, if at all. Saldaña (1999, p. 66) proposes the following options for how a researcher may appear in the ethnodramatic text: "1. a leading role 2. an extra not commenting, just reacting 3. a servant 4. the lead's best friend 5. an offstage voice heard on speakers 6. a character cut from the play in an earlier draft." These are examples and not meant to serve as an exhaustive list. Ultimately, Saldaña suggests that the level of overt analysis and interpretation depends on what is necessary for the promotion of audience understanding. In addition to facilitating understanding, a common goal in the (re)presentation stage, the place of the researcher in the ethnodramatic script is inextricably linked to the epistemological and theoretical underpinning of the study. For example, scholars working from "power-reflexive" or "power-sensitive" perspectives (Haraway, 1991; Pfohl, 1994) such as critical theory, queer studies, feminism, critical race theory, postcolonialism, poststructuralism, and postmodernism may be particularly attentive to how power operates in part via the researcher's choices with respect to disclosure and authority. Scholars working from interpretive traditions or feminist epistemological positions may be particularly concerned with the plane on which researcher and participant operate and how that is communicated to an audience in a full and authentic way.

Characters and their dialogue are one part of script construction. As with all plays, ethnodramas are scripted stories and follow conventions of plot, storyline, and structure. In other words, what is the narrative being communicated? Although the terms "plot" and "storyline" are commonly used synonymously, Saldaña (2003) clarifies these terms for a nontheater audience, defining *plot* as the overall play structure and *storyline* as the progression or sequence of events within the plot. Unlike conventional playwriting, in the construction of ethnodramas, plotting and storylining begin as distinct processes but eventually become interlinked processes (2003, p. 220). Saldaña (2005) notes that *plotting* is the "conceptual framework of ethnodrama" (p. 15).

In addition to plot and storyline, the structures that frame the play also communicate meaning. Typically called "units" in theater, traditional structures include acts, scenes, and vignettes that may be arranged in a linear or episodic sequence (Saldaña, 2003). How the story unfolds will depend on the analytic process the data have undergone and the range of meanings the researcher intends to convey. In accord with ethical praxis, it may be important to find clear ways to disclose the researcher's interpretive role within the script-building process—regardless of, although interlinked with, what kind of character the researcher embodies in the script.

Differing from research findings presented in traditional textual forms, performed ethnodramas also have a visual dimension. In this way, performance pieces allow researchers to capture and communicate the visual components of social life, which are indistinguishable from human experience and our study of it. In particular, scenography communicates information about the time, place, and social climate, while costumes help establish "the look" of the characters and show (Saldaña, 2003, p. 228).

- How have qualitative researchers employed ethnodrama and ethnotheater? What research questions have been explored via these methods?
- How have researchers adapted to the issues reviewed in order to facilitate their own objectives?
- How does collaboration enter into the playwriting and performing processes?
- What is the place of the researcher within these processes? How is reflexivity achieved?
- How can ethnodrama and related methods be used as a means of accessing subjugated perspectives?

Ethnodrama, Health Theater, and Subjugated Voices: Ethical Issues in Practice

One field in which ethnodrama has emerged as an important alternative method is health studies. In this area, drama is a vehicle for communicating the experiences of sick people. Mienczakowski, Smith, and Morgan (2002) use ethnodrama to create *health theater*, which refers to performed ethnodramas that focus on health-related issues. The ethical issues that surface in all ethnodramatic research become particularly pronounced in health theater, and these researchers suggest that while practitioners attempt to execute their own agendas, they must be vigilant against potential harmful effects on audience members. In one empirical study Mienczakowski and colleagues developed a health theater performance based on interviews conducted with people diagnosed with schizophrenia. The show, titled "Syncing Out Loud" (Mienczakowksi, 1994), enabled the audience to learn about the experience of this particular illness from the perspective of the research participants who live with it. In this way, the researchers report that the performance both confronted and dispelled misconceptions and prejudices associated with this disease and mental disorders in general. Based on their experience in this area, Mienczakowski and colleagues assert that a performance-based methodology within health studies creates a space for the voices of marginalized health-care recipients and caregivers (professional and personal). Ethnotheater can thus be used to access and present subjugated voices, to educate, and to confront and work through stereotypes and misunderstandings. Moreover, ethnotheater has the potential to emancipate (Mienczakowski, 1995).

Even though this method carries these positive social justice–oriented possibilities, there are also potential pitfalls, and as such Mienczakowski and colleagues (2002) argue for guidelines for the ethical practice of health theater. Health theater is a form of public performance; therefore, the researchers bear responsibility for the impact of the performance on audience well-being, just as qualitative researchers have an obligation to protect their informants' confidentiality and to leave informants and their environment unharmed (see Bailey, 1996, 2007). The need to create guidelines specific to this method has arisen from incidents in which audience members were put at risk as a result of witnessing an ethnodramatic performance. For example, Mienczakowski and colleagues cite the example of two attempted suicides after a performance titled "Tears in the Shadows." The strategies they propose can also be employed to add dimensions of validity to a study, thus serving a dual purpose.

Mienczakowski and colleagues propose two particular strategies. First, they suggest having a preview performance of the drama for an audience with knowledge about the topic under investigation. Second, "post-performance forum sessions" can be used to analyze audience responses to assess the show's impact (2002, p. 49). In these ways, as researchers navigate the ethical issues that emerge with this form of inquiry, so too have they created measures for maximizing validity and trustworthiness.

Conquergood (1985) identifies four additional ethical mistakes researchers working with performance-based methods can make, particularly when trying to (re)present subjugated perspectives. The mistakes he notes are: (1) making a sacred text no longer sacred, (2) failing to connect to the text or performance, (3) denying the possible tense nature of sensitive material, and (4) sensationalizing cultural differences (1985, p. 4). Attention to these ethical issues is also a part of creating authenticity.

Performance Ethnography and Reflexivity

In addition to serving as a method for investigating and representing the experiences and perspectives of various groups, performance ethnography can also serve as a vehicle for addressing the research process itself, that is, how the knowledge-building process unfolds, including how it is experienced by the researcher and others involved. In this regard, an excellent example comes from Laurie Thorp's (2003) research titled "Voices From the Garden: A Performance Ethnography."

Thorp's (2003) project began as her doctoral fieldwork in agricultural education. Although the research comes in part from the ethnographic research she conducted (with nearly 150 children and eight teachers), it also chronicles her personal and professional experience during the research process. For example, while working on the study she was confronted with her father's death, and thus her grieving process is entwined with her experience of cocreating this knowledge. Moreover, Thorp documents her experiences working with an "emergent research method" or innovative methods practice (see Hesse-Biber & Leavy, 2006), and how others involved in the process, including her dissertation advisor, helped her navigate the process and modify her perceptions as necessary in order to reveal insight that would not have been possible within a different methodological framework.

The cast and set are as follows: Six stools are on stage arranged in a semicircle. The characters, or "readers," are: Laurie Thorp, an elementary school teacher; an elementary school student; the dissertation advisor (renowned methodologist Yvonna S. Lincoln); a university student volunteer (Daniel Brooks); and the Poet Muse. Behind the six readers there are projected photographic images from the garden, and objects from the garden are placed at the foot of the stools. The house lights are dimmed, with soft lights on the six readers. Focusing on Thorp herself, the dissertation advisor, and the Poet Muse as the three "characters" that allow for the greatest overt analysis and interpretation of the knowledge-building process itself, some excerpts from the script follow:

> DISSERTATION ADVISOR: "Write your way through this darkness; you have a story to tell." (p. 314)
>
> POET MUSE: "Voice is meaning that resides in the individual and enables that individual to participate in community." (p. 316)
>
> DISSERTATION ADVISOR: "I might add that as Laurie relinquished control of the inquiry process, she came much closer to what is 'really real' at this school than any research objectives or proposal could ever anticipate." (p. 318)
>
> LAURIE: "Hold on to your hearts; I've saved the best for last. They don't get any better than this. This is what makes research so damn rewarding. Just when you least expect it, the data jump out at you with a showstopper. And I can really toot the horn on this one 'cause I didn't figure it out, nope, not me. I puzzled and puzzled, cogitated and analyzed, and finally yelled uncle. So I met up for dinner one night with Gloria (*points to teacher*) and said, 'Help, what does all of this mean?' She nearly took my breath away with her powers of insight and interpretation." (p. 322)

As you can see, these particular voices serve the script by making explicit the struggles—personal, epistemological, theoretical, practical, and so forth—that come to bear on the meaning-making process. In this way, the script chronicles the meaning-making process itself from the perspective of the researcher struggling through it, but in conversation with the literature about knowledge-building. The conclusion of the script begins as follows:

> DISSERTATION ADVISOR: "Laurie, I see our time is drawing to a close, but before we conclude, would you share some of the 'lessons learned' from this, your journey of a lifetime?"
>
> LAURIE: "I must say that I'm a bit uneasy these days with recommending anything to anyone. Yet Clifford Geertz has said that as we traverse from 'being there' to 'being here,' we somehow must find a place to stand. So, here is where I stand, for the time being: Open yourself to emergent design, emergent learning, emergent planning. Go ahead, let it

unfold. I promise you won't be disappointed. It is liberating; you can't imagine what you will hear, what you will learn, and most important, what you will do.

"While you are there, stay awhile. Stay a long while. Prolonged engagement pays dividends, big dividends, in currency rarely traded these days: care, commitment, and human understanding.

"While you are waiting, be sure to reflect. And reflect out loud so we can all hear, I really mean it. Our closed system of discourse needs to reflexively come clean regarding our politics, our ethics, our ways of knowing, and all the other entanglements that occur in all research settings. Reflexivity acknowledges my vulnerability and I like that, for I am tired of the smooth, shiny certainty found in most academic journals.

"We hold the power of legitimized knowledge production in academia; make something happen. Don't become complacent with your privilege. Go ahead, you pick; there are hundreds of untold stories out there waiting to be told ...

(*Laurie stands and moves to front and center*) "There is a lump in my throat today that reminds me of the many difficult good-byes I've known in my life. ... I am a daughter writing my self through grief. I am a woman writing my self into being ... " (p. 323)

As evidenced by these powerful excerpts, this methodology allows researchers to reflexively investigate the research process itself, and how we move within it, as well as diverse subject matter.

- What other performance-based methods do researchers employ?

Performative Mapping

The use of multiple voices within the script-building process also occurs with the method of *performative mapping,* which is a collage-style performance that occurs through performed dialogue. Daspit and McDermott (2002) presented data at a conference via performative mapping, a fluid method of representation. Furthermore, Daspit and McDermott explain that the appeal of arts-based practices in general lies in their ability to facilitate looking at data in new ways. When constructing their piece they embed each piece of the collage, or each "scrap," with particular significance that is stitched together in order to create meaning. They write:

> Of course performances are inherently re-presentational, and re-representations are always performances. But the in-between "space" of performance and re-presentation creates an experiential, aesthetic heuristic we call "performative mapping." (p. 179)

The nature of (re)presentation and performance is what draws some scholars to this methodological genre.

Robert E. Rinehart (2005) created a performance text because of the synchronicity between the method and topic of his study. Rinehart wrote a four-act play with the aim of showing how contemporary sports are about performance, creating a shift in the sports arena. The dialogue consisted of different voices/narrators from the sports world such as players, workers, and audience members. The message repeated throughout the play, with respect to content and form and via the different voices, is that in contemporary culture the art of sport centers on performance.

Theater Arts and Education

Drama is employed in education and social research as a methodological tool for educational training purposes as well as other issues surrounding teaching and learning. In this area many of the techniques employed within the theater arts, such as role-playing, improvisation, and skits, come to bear in educational research.

Matthew J. Meyer (2004) evaluated "theater as representation," referred to as TAR, as a method for educator training. Meyer used data collected from interviews with current educators and administrators to determine which dimensions of educator training he wanted to access, and then used what he gleaned from the interview data to develop a series of theater-based methods, including role-playing, skits, case-study participation, leadership games, and simulations. Meyer reports that the project was successful and that TAR helped better prepare educators because the methods facilitate hands-on learning. Moreover, these hands-on methods expand self reflection during the process (p. 7).

Rogers, Frellick, and Babinski (2002) also employed theater as a representational form in their research aimed at assisting teachers. Rogers and colleagues designed a study with the intent of exploring the problems that first-year teachers encounter. The study was conducted in North Carolina from 1995 to 2000, during which the researchers facilitated 19 discussion groups of 100 new teachers divided into groups of three to nine participants who met twice a week to discuss solving problems they were experiencing in the classroom. Initially the researchers represented the data in a traditional report; however, they found that format ineffective in conveying the emotion of the groups and their authentic messages and themes. Rogers and colleagues write, "We found this process and its final product to be empty, lifeless, and extremely unsatisfying" (p. 53). In an attempt to find a form that was compatible with what they wanted to impart, Rogers and colleagues tried drama and found it to be an effective representational form for conveying ideas, emotions, and messages in a way that invited outsiders to identify the key issues and address them in discussions afterwards. They note "immediacy" as one of the advantages of TAR. Moreover, they refer to their final work as a "moving piece" that contains the potential to instigate change and discussion in the teaching field.

The example of Rogers and colleagues (2002) extends beyond the usefulness of theater as a representational form and serves as a lesson about working with new arts-based practices. Researchers who experiment with these methods often have to be willing to modify their research, acknowledge when a traditional form isn't working, and take a methodological risk in an attempt to serve their project.

- How can performance pieces be evaluated? What criteria are used to judge performances? What strategies are available for adding validity and authenticity into the (re)presentation of the data?
- How are audience members involved in the evaluative process? How is this process collaborative?

Issues of Validity, Authenticity, and Assessment

In performance-based research, standards of validity and assessment center on the issue of *authenticity*. Throughout this chapter some of the measures available for achieving validity have been addressed in relation to other aspects of performance-based research. Here I cogently revisit some of these strategies and propose additional ones. It is important to bear in mind that issues of authenticity and validity are linked to the research purpose in a given project, as well as to the researcher's theoretical framework.

As noted earlier, Saldaña (1999) proposes strategies for building validity into the script-construction process (i.e., he suggests how to design a study with validity checks built in to the data collection and analysis phases). Specifically, Saldaña proposes variations on *triangulation* as data is selected, *highlighting disconfirming data,* and *exhibiting collective story creation* (which means dialogue has occurred consistently) (p. 64).

J. Cho and Allen Trent (2005), in proposing several strategies for how performance-based research can be assessed, ultimately suggest a mix of methods. Cho and Trent create their validity checks by adapting some of the issues raised by Conquergood's (1985) research on "dialogical performance" and Madison's (2003) "possibilities performance."

Dialogical performance involves a dialogue between different people or researchers and texts. This method enables multiple views, new ideas, and a renegotiation of ideas. In this regard Cho and Trent write, "Dialogical performance theory seeks an open-ended, co-existential, intimate, honest, courageous understanding between self and other" (2005, p. 3).

Madison's "possibilities performance" creates a space where possibilities can be actualized. In this framework marginalized voices can emerge (via characters), allowing the audience to see possibilities for how the social world can change. Ideally, such an experience motivates audience members to be a part of positive social progress.

These dialectical methods of performance prompt discussion that gives the audience a glimpse into their roles (and how they could be configured differently), and allows silenced persons a space for expression. Therefore, building on these performance theories, Cho and Trent (2005) advocate preperformance, performance, and postperformance stages of discussion/feedback. During the preperformance discussion, the data collected can be used to create or alter the script. During the performance there is an exchange between the performers and audience. The "success" of the performance is based on the perceived *authenticity* of the text and the *aesthetics* of the performance. Finally, the postperformance stage allows the researcher to prompt a dialogue where ideas are struggled over. In this final stage the researcher assesses the effect of the performance on the audience. Norris (2000) also proposes that dramatic performance stimulates discussion with the audience, allowing for the continued negotiation of meaning. Norris writes:

> This makes the process recursive as our research dissemination also becomes a means of data collection. It is a form of participatory research where the text ceases to be a declarative authorial one but one in which consumers can become producers and vice versa. (p. 48)

In performance studies, the data collected during and after the representational stage, when traditional research has typically ended, becomes another measure of validity.

In performance-based research the "success" of the performance is intimately linked to the research purpose. For example, if the goal of the research was to access subjugated perspectives, how well did the performance accomplish this? If raising consciousness and awareness was a goal of the study, how well was that accomplished based on postperformance discussion, interviews, focus groups, or surveys? Denzin (2006) suggests that we consider the following questions, as they relate to our study: Does the performance nurture a critical race consciousness? Does the performance heal or empower? Does the performance represent a "pedagogy of hope"? Does the performance subvert and critique official ideology? Does the study avoid ethical landmines? Is a feminist or otherwise social justice–oriented ethic enacted? Answering these questions is how we can address issues of validity, trustworthiness, and authenticity in the context of performance studies.

Checklist of Considerations

✓ What is the goal of the study, and how does performance serve the goal?

✓ Will the entire structure of the research design be dramatic, or will drama serve as a data collection form or representational form only?

✓ How will the data be obtained (ethnography, interview, public documents, etc.)? What performance-based method will be employed? Is this method collaborative?

✓ During script construction how will plot, narrative, and overall structure be conceived? How will characters be created? What validity checks am I using to ensure three-dimensional portrayals? How will dialogue and monologue be generated? What ethical issues might emerge?

✓ How do I deal with disconfirming data? What procedures for yielding authenticity and validity will be employed? What procedures for postshow dialogue will be used?

Conclusion

This chapter has served as an introduction to performance studies. This is an expansive interdisciplinary methodological genre with the potential to continue to cultivate epistemological, theoretical, and methodological innovation. In the following reading Diane Conrad offers an empirical example of her work using the method of *Popular Theatre,* a participatory performance ethnography method. Conrad employed Popular Theatre in a study of how high school drama students in a rural community perceived the ways in which their life experiences and opportunities were affected by their environment. The performance-based method ultimately allowed both the research participants and the researcher to reexamine their assumptions and beliefs. Conrad argues that Popular Theatre is an effective research method and pedagogical tool.

DISCUSSION QUESTIONS AND ACTIVITIES

1. What are the similarities between the craft of qualitative research and the practice of drama and theater arts? How can these similarities be harnessed to produce rich qualitative research?

2. What are the primary research purposes served by performance-based methods?

3. What are the primary performance-based research methods? What is distinct about each method?

4. How can performance research be assessed? What research design issues need consideration with respect to validity and authenticity?

5. For this exercise, select a research topic (e.g., body image, sexual identity, youth killings) and collect a sample of data from public sources (including an academic literature review). How might you begin coding or cataloguing this data with the intent of creating a performance script? Note how themes, characters, dialogue, and narrative begin to emerge. For a variation on this activity, work in a small group of three to five people and follow this same process with the goal of "collective creation."

SUGGESTED READINGS

Denzin, N. K. (2003). *Performance ethnography: Critical pedagogy and the politics of culture.* Thousand Oaks, CA: Sage.

This advanced book covers performance ethnography from critical perspectives. The book reviews topics such as postmodernism, performance as critical pedagogy, and ethics.

Madison, D. S. (2005). *Critical ethnography: Method, ethics, and performance.* Thousand Oaks, CA: Sage.

This is a sophisticated review of critical ethnography and performance that covers complex theoretical issues and methods while providing empirical examples.

Madison, D. S., & Hamera, J. (Eds.). (2006). *The Sage handbook of performance studies.* Thousand Oaks, CA: Sage.

This handbook provides a comprehensive retrospective and prospective review of performance studies, with theoretical chapters as well as contributions based on empirical research. In general, the chapters are advanced and appropriate for researchers, scholars, and graduate students.

Saldaña, J. (Ed.). (2005). *Ethnodrama: An anthology of reality theater.* Walnut Creek, CA: AltaMira Press.

This edited volume provides an outstanding collection of ethnodramas, all written in dramatic form. The contents are divided into three sections: ethnodramatic monologue, ethnodramatic dialogue with monologue, and ethnodramatic extensions. The appendix in the back of the book is a fantastic resource that offers suggested readings categorized by the different dramatic model employed in the study (e.g., autoethnography models, narrator as a key figure).

Schechner, R. (2002). *Performance studies: An introduction.* New York: Routledge.

This comprehensive book provides a perspective on the nuts and bolts of performance studies.

SUGGESTED WEBSITES AND JOURNALS

International Journal of Performance Arts and Digital Media
    www.intellectbooks.co.uk/journals.appx.php?issn=14794713

The *International Journal of Performance Arts and Digital Media* is a new interdisciplinary peer-reviewed journal drawing contributions from diverse researchers and practitioners who work at the interface of new technologies and performance arts.

Studies in Theatre and Performance
    www.ovid.com/site/catalog/Journal/2452.jsp?top=2&mid=3&bottom=7&subsection=12

Studies in Theatre and Performance is a new multidisciplinary peer-reviewed journal for scholars, teachers, and practitioners to publish methodological, theoretical, and empirical research in the area of theater practice, as well as work with regard to teaching and performance. This journal serves as the official publication for the Standing Conference of University Drama Departments in the United Kingdom.

REFERENCES

Bailey, C. (1996). *A guide to field research.* Thousand Oaks, CA: Pine Forge Press.

Bailey, C. (2007). *A guide to qualitative field research.* Thousand Oaks, CA: Pine Forge Press.

Berry, G., & Reinbold, J. (1984). *Collective creation.* Edmonton, AL, Canada: Alberta Alcohol and Drug Abuse Commission.

Bhabha, H. (1993). Culture's in between. *Artform International, 32*(1), 167–171.

Butler, J. (1993). Critically queer. *GLQ: A Journal of Gay and Lesbian Studies, 1,* 17–32.

Charmaz, K. (2008). Grounded theory as an emergent method. In S. N. Hesse-Biber & P. Leavy (Eds), *Handbook of emergent methods* (pp. 155–170). New York: Guilford Press.

Cho, J., & Trent, A. (2005). *Process-based validity for performance-related qualitative work: Imaginative, artistic, and co-reflexive criteria.* Pullman: Washington State University.

Conquergood, D. (1985). Performing as a moral act: Ethical dimensions of the ethnography of performance. *Literature in Performance, 5,* 1–13.

Daspit, T., & McDermott, M. (2002). Frameworks of blood and bone: An alchemy of performative mapping. In C. Bagley & M. B. Cancienne (Eds), *Dancing the data* (pp. 177–190). New York: Peter Lang.

Denzin, N. K. (1997). *Interpretive ethnography: Ethnographic practices for the 21st century.* Thousand Oaks, CA: Sage.

Denzin, N. K. (2006). The politics and ethics of performance pedagogy: Toward a pedagogy of hope. In D. S. Madison & J. Hamera (Eds.), *The Sage handbook of performance studies* (pp. 325–338). Thousand Oaks, CA: Sage.

Donmoyer, R., & Yennie-Donmoyer, J. (1995). Data as drama: Reflections on the use of Readers' Theatre as a mode of qualitative data display. *Qualitative Inquiry, 1,* 402–428.

Finley, S. (1998, April). *Traveling through the cracks: Homeless youth speak out.* Paper performed at the annual meeting of the American Education Research Association, San Diego, CA.

Frisch, M. (1990). *A shared authority: Essays on the craft and meaning of oral and public history.* Albany: State University of New York Press.

Goffman, E. (1959). *The presentation of self in everyday life.* Garden City, NY: Anchor.

Gray, R. E. (2003). Performing on and off the stage: The place(s) of performance in arts-based approaches to qualitative inquiry. *Qualitative Inquiry, 9*(2), 254–267.

Haraway, D. (1991). *Simians, cyborgs, and women: The reinvention of nature.* New York: Routledge.

Hesse-Biber, S. N., & Leavy, P. (2006). *Emergent methods in social research.* Thousand Oaks, CA: Sage.

Langellier, K. M., & Peterson, E. E. (2006). Shifting contexts in personal narrative performance. In D. S. Madison & J. Hamera (Eds.), *The Sage handbook of performance studies* (pp. 151–168). Thousand Oaks, CA: Sage.

Lincoln, Y. S. (2004). Performing 9/11: Teaching in a terrorized world. *Qualitative Inquiry, 10*(1), 140–159.

Madison, D. S. (2003). Performance, personal narrative, and the politics of possibility. In Y. Lincoln & N. Denzin (Eds.), *Turning points in qualitative research* (pp. 469–486). New York: AltaMira Press.

McLeod, J. (1988). *The arts and education.* Paper presented at an invitational seminar cosponsored by the Fine Arts Council of the Alberta Teachers' Association and the University of Alberta, Faculty of Education, Edmonton, Alberta, Canada.

Meyer, M. J. (2004). Theater as representation (TAR) in the teaching of teacher and administrator preparation programs. *International Electronic Journal for Leadership in Learning, 8*(6), 1–21.

Mienczakowski, J. (1994). *Syncing out loud: A journey into illness* (2nd ed.). Brisbane, Australia: Griffith University.

Mienczakowski, J. (1995). The theater of ethnography: The reconstruction of ethnography into theater with emancipatory potential. *Qualitative Inquiry, 1,* 360–375.

Mienczakowski, J., Smith, L., & Morgan, S. (2002). Seeing words—Hearing feelings: Ethnodrama and the performance of data. In C. Bagley & M. B. Cancienne (Eds.), *Dancing the data* (pp. 90–104). New York: Peter Lang.

Moreira, C. (2005, May). *Made for sex.* Paper presented at the First International Congress of Qualitative Inquiry, Urbana–Champaign, IL.

Norris, J. (2000). Drama as research: Realizing the potential of drama in education as a research methodology. *Youth Theatre Journal, 14,* pp. 40–51.

Oikarinen-Jabai, H. (2003). Toward performative research: Embodied listening to the self/other. *Qualitative Inquiry, 9*(4), 569–579.

Pfohl, S. (1994). *Images of deviance and social control: A sociological history.* New York: McGraw-Hill.

Rinehart, R. E. (2005). *Sports performance in four acts: Players, workers, audience, and immortality.* Pullman: Washington State University.

Rogers, D., Frellick, P., & Babinski, L. (2002). Staging a study: Performing the personal and professional struggles of beginning teachers. In C. Bagley & M. B. Cancienne (Eds.), *Dancing the data* (pp. 53–69). New York: Peter Lang.

Saldaña, J. (1998). *Ethical issues in an ethnographic performance text: The "dramatic impact" of "juicy stuff."* Tempe: Arizona State University Press.

Saldaña, J. (1999). Playwriting with data: Ethnographic performance texts. *Youth Theatre Journal, 14,* 60–71.

Saldaña, J. (Ed.). (2005). *Ethnodrama: An anthology of reality theater.* Walnut Creek, CA: AltaMira Press.

Saldaña, J. (2003). Dramatizing data: A primer. *Qualitative Inquiry, 9*(2), 218–236.

Tarlington, C., & Michaels, W. (1995). *Building plays: Simple playbuilding techniques at work.* Markham, ON, Canada: Pembroke.

Thorp, L. (2003). Voices from the garden: A performance ethnography. *Qualitative Inquiry, 9*(2), 312–324.

Turner, V. (1974). *Drama, fields, and metaphors: Symbolic action in human society.* Ithaca, NY: Routledge.

Valentine, K. B. (2006). Unlocking the doors for incarcerated women through performance and creative writing. In D. S. Madison & J. Hamera (Eds.), *The Sage handbook of performance studies* (pp. 309–324). Thousand Oaks, CA: Sage.

Warren, B. (1993). *Using the creative arts in therapy: A practical introduction.* New York: Routledge.

Worthen, W. B. (1998). Drama, performativity, and performance. *PMLA, 133*(5), 1093–1107.

Exploring Risky Youth Experiences

Popular Theatre as a Participatory, Performative Research Method

Diane Conrad

For my doctoral research, I wanted to better understand the experiences of youth from their perspective, in particular the kinds of experiences that might deem them "at risk." In prior work with so-called "at-risk" youth in inner-city high schools, a young offender facility, a youth drop-in center, and in two Northwest Territories communities, youth had often told me that they found the label "at-risk" offensive.

The label is commonly used in education to talk about students "at-risk" of failing or dropping out of school, in health care regarding youths' lifestyle choices detrimental to their mental or physical health, and in criminal justice with respect to the risk of their involvement with the criminal justice system. Discourse around "at-risk," however, seems largely based on the logics of economics, a fear that "at-risk" youth will not become productive and contributing members of society. Risk factors used to describe "at-risk" youth or predict who might be "at risk," are based on a deficit model, portraying youth, their families, and their communities as somehow deficient or deviant if they do not meet society's expectations (National Coalition of Advocates for Students, 1985).

I wanted to better understand the implications for youth labeled "at-risk." To this end, I planned to engage a group of high school drama students in exploring issues they identified as relevant to their lives through a Popular Theatre process. The rural Alberta community in which I conducted my research had, as it turned out, a majority aboriginal population. Statistically, I knew that I was likely to find fewer so-called "at-risk" youth in predominantly white, middle-class urban or suburban schools. As my previous research had been in an inner-city context, I opted for a rural Alberta setting this time. I did not seek to work with aboriginal youth specifically, but when the predicament of aboriginal youth in Alberta presented itself, I was unwilling to evade it. As I was to learn, aboriginal youth in Alberta are among those most often labeled "at-risk" of dropping out of school (Alberta Learning, 2001).[1] I use the inclusive term "aboriginal" in my research to refer youth belonging to racial/cultural groups indigenous to the Alberta region where I worked, and for ethical reasons as the predicament of "at-risk" youth extends beyond any one particular group.

My study explored the potential of Popular Theatre as a pedagogical tool and a research methodology, as the drama students and I enacted it. As this article illustrates, Popular Theatre draws on traditions in both participatory (Fals-Borda & Rahman, 1991; Kidd & Byram, 1978; McTaggart, 1997; Park, Brydon-Miller, Hall, & Jackson, 1993) and arts-based/performed ethnographic approaches (Conquergood, 1998; Fabian, 1990; Turner, 1986) as an effective means of collectively drawing out and examining participants' experiences toward producing new understandings. Popular Theatre, as a qualitative research method that is both participatory and performative, presents alternative ways to engage participants in doing research.

This article focuses on Popular Theatre as a research method. Following the Popular Theatre phase of my research process, I wrote a series of *scripted descriptions* depicting significant moments from the participatory work with students, an example of which is included. I drew on these scripts to engage in a reflective, interpretive process including discourse analysis and autoethnographic inquiry to help me make sense of what the Popular Theatre work with students revealed. I begin here by making theoretical links between Popular Theatre and other methodological approaches, and then discuss the Popular Theatre project with students, which we entitled "Life in the Sticks."

What Is *Popular Theatre?*

The term *Popular Theatre* was used by Canadian Ross Kidd (among others) in the 1970s to talk about the form of development work he was doing in Botswana and Zimbabwe at the time (Kidd, 1982). Popular Theatre[2] is "a process of theatre which deeply involves specific communities in identifying issues of concern, analyzing current conditions and causes of a situation, identifying points of change, and analyzing how change could happen and/or contributing to the actions implied" (Prentki & Selman, 2000, p. 8). Better defined by its intentions of personal and social transformation than by the various forms it may take, Popular Theatre draws on participants' experiences to collectively create theater and engage in discussion of issues through theatrical means.

The work of Bertolt Brecht in 1930s Germany was a theatrical form that influenced the development of Western Popular Theatre in the way it reclaimed theater for political and community functions. Brecht felt that realism in the theater encouraged passivity among bourgeois audiences, suppressing the inclination to be active participants in the theater as in life. Brecht looked for ways to break the theatrical "fourth wall," in order to raise awareness amongst his audiences. His Epic Theatre used techniques of "alienation" within the dramatic action, including episodic scenes interrupted by narration, songs, parables, the projection of texts and images, to break the illusion of the performance and to make audiences active interpreters of the multilayered text rather than playing on their emotions. For Brecht, Epic Theatre "appeals less to the feelings than to the spectator's reason. Instead of sharing the experience the spectator must come to grips with things" (1957/1964, p. 23). The Epic Theatre experience awoke a critical consciousness in the spectator.

In the 1960s and 1970s, Popular Theatre grew out of the popular education movement, with Paulo Freire of Brazil being one of popular education's best known proponents. Freire developed his *Pedagogy of the Oppressed* (1970) in a time of extreme political repression in Brazil. His liberatory literacy education involved not only reading the *word*, but also reading the *world* through the development of critical consciousness or conscientization. A critical consciousness allowed people to question the nature of their historical and social situation—to *read* their world—with the goal of acting as subjects in the creation of a democratic society. Like Brecht, Freire too wanted human beings to take an active role in their lives. His popular education methods countered the dominant system of education—a system inherently oppressive and dehumanizing that he described as a "banking model"—where students were passive recipients of the teacher's knowledge.

Popular education programs with similar goals developed around the same time, and still continue, particularly in adult education and community development projects around the world.[3] Popular education is aimed at empowering traditionally excluded, marginalized, or subordinated sectors of society. With the political intentions of collective social change toward a more equitable and democratic society through raised awareness and collaborative action, popular education practices explore the learners' lived experiences in both their humanizing and oppressive dimensions. It draws on and validates learners' knowledge in the production of new knowledge. Through critical dialogue, reflection, and problem posing, learners discuss the possibilities of transforming the oppressive elements of their experience culminating in collective social action. This involves a dynamic of reflection and action or "praxis" (Freire, 1970), a concept central to participatory processes.

In the 1960s, inspired by Brecht's theatrical techniques and Freire's popular education approach, Augusto Boal, another Brazilian, developed a specific set of theatrical techniques he called the *Theatre of the Oppressed* (1979).[4] Like Brecht, his theater challenged traditional theatrical conventions. For Boal, the commercial or professional theater was an instrument of the ruling class, creating divisions in society by separating the actor from the spectator. In traditional theater, the spectator is invited to identify and empathize with the characters in the drama, and the play provides, at its end, an Aristotelian sense of catharsis, leaving the spectator with a feeling of resolution, a fundamentally passive exercise. To create active audiences, Boal's theater not only breaks the "fourth wall" but also the division between actor and audience by transforming the spectator into a "spect-actor" by taking on the role of the protagonist. His techniques of Image Theatre, Simultaneous Dramaturgy, and Forum Theatre give the audience a part in the dramatic action, by discussing plans for change, directing the action, and/or trying out different solutions through drama. For Boal, *Theatre of the Oppressed* was a weapon for oppressed people to use toward changing their social reality—theater for the people, by the people, "a rehearsal of revolution" (1974/1979, p. 155).

Following his arrest, torture, and exile from Brazil for his political involvements, Boal went to Europe where he continued his work. To meet the needs of his European participants, who felt more anxious and alienated than oppressed, his *Rainbow of Desire* (1995) took a more therapeutic or psychodramatic approach based on his belief that "to revolutionize society requires both an analytical overview of social history and a personal, practical investigation of one's own behavioural psychology" (Cohen-Cruz & Schutzman, 1994, p. 145). On his return to Rio de Janeiro and subsequent election to Brazilian parliament in 1993, Boal developed techniques of Legislative Theatre (1999), a method of consulting the public on government issues through theater.

Popular Theatre as Participatory Research

In the 1970s, in association with the popular education movement, participatory research developed around the world as a research method

(Fals-Borda & Rahman, 1991; Freire, 1988; McTaggart, 1997; Park et al., 1993).[5]

Viewed both as a means of creating knowledge and as a tool for education, the development of consciousness and mobilization for action, participatory research involves a process of "transformative praxis" (Fals-Borda & Rahman, 1991). As research "for," "with," and "by" the people rather than "on" the people, it seeks to break down the distinction between researchers and researched—the subject–object relationship of traditional research instead creating a subject–subject relationship. Ideally, participants are involved in the research process from beginning to end, in the attainment, creation, and dissemination of knowledge. Participatory research stresses the inherent capacity for participants to create their own knowledge based on their experiences. In the process, "popular knowledge" is generated by the group, taken in, analyzed, and reaffirmed or criticized, making it possible to flesh out a problem and understand it in context.

Striving to end the monopoly of the written word, participatory research has traditionally incorporated alternative methods, including photography, radio, poetry, music, myths, drawing, sculpture, puppets, and Popular Theatre, as meeting spaces for cultural exchange. Drawing on an affective logic involving sentiment and emotions rather than purely scientific logic, the group process ceases to convey isolated opinions as with surveys or interviews—becoming instead a springboard for collective reasoning. The knowledge produced is socially heard, legitimized, and added to the people's collective knowledge, empowering them to solve their own problems (Fals-Borda & Rahman, 1991). For Salazar (1991), participatory research is more than just a research method; it is "an egalitarian philosophy of life designed to break unjust or exploitative power relations and to achieve a more satisfactory kind of society" (p. 62).

Popular Theatre, as a method of participatory research, involves shared ownership of the research process and community-based analysis of issues, all with an orientation toward community action.

Popular Theatre as Performative Research

Popular Theatre as a research method builds on qualitative methods, such as Clandinin and Connelly's (2000) narrative inquiry, and alternative or arts-based ways of knowing and representing research (Diamond & Mullen, 1999; Eisner, 1997; Finley, 2003). A postmodern attitude toward "truth" and the production of knowledge has legitimized an abundance of alternative approaches to doing research and new forms of representing research in the social sciences.[6] Among these, arts-based researchers have written performative texts, performed their research, and used performance to gather participant responses and interpret them (Conrad, 2002; Norris, 2000; Saldaña, 2003). Denzin calls ethnodrama "the single most powerful way for ethnography to recover yet interrogate the meanings of lived experience" (1997, p. 94) and elsewhere calls for research that is pedagogical, political, and performative (2003).

Performative research or performance ethnography has roots in the fields of anthropology (Fabian, 1990; Turner, 1986) and communication/performance studies (Conquergood, 1998), where performance is regarded as both a legitimate and an ethical way of representing ethnographic understanding. In their research, performance ethnographers find or create opportunities to perform their cultural understandings by observing, participating in performances, and/or representing their findings to others through performance. As instances of performance that provide cultural understanding, performance ethnographers inquire into cultural events: public occasions, rituals, games, storytelling, theater, and dance; social dramas or dramatic events in everyday life such as moments of conflict; everyday interactions including culturally conditioned behavior, the performance of social roles of gender, race, status, age, and so on; and communicative/speech acts that are performative (Austin, 1975; Butler, 1997). In performance ethnography, performance spills from the stage into "real" life.

Recently, the notion of performance (or performativity) has been taken up by qualitative social researchers as a form of critical pedagogy in doing arts-based inquiry (Finley, 2003), in the writing of performance texts (Denzin, 2003), and in critical arts education (Garoian, 1999). For Denzin, performance ethnography as praxis is "a way of acting on the world in order to change it" (2003, p. 228). Finley asserts that performance creates an open, dialogic space for inquiry and expression through "an imaginative interpretation of events and the contexts of their occurrences" (p. 287). For Garoian (1999), performance opens a liminal pedagogical space that allows for a reflexive learning process that "recognize[s] the cultural experiences, memories, and perspectives—participants' multiple voices—as viable content ... encourages participant discussions of complex and contradictory issues" (p. 67) and includes the involvement of the observer. As a passionate, visceral, and kinetic activity, performance creates opportunities for communion among participants, researchers, and research audiences.

In Popular Theatre, participants' performances depict and examine their "performances" in real life, providing insight into their lived experiences and their cultural world. As Fabian claims, some types of cultural knowledge cannot simply be called up and expressed in discursive statements by informants, but can be represented "only through action, enactment, or performance" (1990, p. 6). Knowledge of culture or social life is performative rather than informative. In this way, Fabian, an anthropologist, pushes insight about performance "toward its methodological imperative: performance as a method, as well as a subject of ethnographic research" (p. 86). In a performative epistemology, performance is an embodied, empathic way of knowing and "deeply sensing the other" (Conquergood, 1985, p. 3).

Popular Theatre makes use of a participatory form of critical performance ethnography, deliberately creating opportunities for exploration through performance or "acting out." What better way to study lived experience than by reenacting it? A Popular Theatre process, which may include drama activities such as image work, improvisation, role-play, and collective creation, engages participants in generating, interpreting, and re-presenting their ideas. By taking on a role, the player exists simultaneously in two worlds: as a character inside the experience of the "as-if" world and as an actor evaluating the situation from the outside, within the real world. The player is both involved and detached, alternating from one to the other observing the self in action, comparing the two worlds to arrive at some understanding or meaning (Courtney, 1988).

Performance theorist Richard Schechner (1985) too sees performance as a paradigm of liminality. Fundamental to all performance is the characteristic of "restored behaviour" or "twice-behaved behaviour" that is "symbolic and reflexive: not empty but loaded behaviour multivocally broadcasting significance ... [in which] the self can act in/as another" (p. 52), allowing individuals to become someone other than themselves. The play frame opens a liminal space where the "not me" encounters the "not-not me" (p. 123). As such, it offers an alternative performative way of knowing—a unique and powerful way of accessing knowledge, drawing out responses that are spontaneous, intuitive, tacit, experiential, embodied, or affective, rather than simply cognitive (Courtney, 1988). In Popular Theatre, through "acting out" participants are involved in a process that is critical and analytic, a mimetic[7] process that has transformative potential (Taussig, 1993).

"Life in the Sticks": A Popular Theatre Project

My doctoral study involving Popular Theatre with a group of high school drama students began from my interest in "at risk," and my search for ways to better meet the educational needs of so-called "at-risk" youth. Popular Theatre was a way for the students and I to collectively examine their experiences for the purposes of raising their awareness (and that of the audiences for which they performed), helping them look for solutions or responses to issues, and to give me insight into their experiences that might deem them "at risk," from their perspective.

With appropriate ethics review board approval, I spent 1 month living and working in the rural Alberta community. The drama teacher at the school was generous in allowing me to work with his two mixed-grade 10–11–12 drama classes during their scheduled class time in the drama room. The group included 22 students in all with an equal number of males and females. Ninety percent of the students at the school were of aboriginal descent, including students of mixed First Nations heritage and of the Métis Nation. The classes I worked with also included some white students. Each class met five times in an 8-day cycle, with each meeting lasting 1 hour, giving us approximately 30 hours of contact time over a 1-month period.

The drama teacher generally included an issues-based component to his program. Some of the students with whom I worked had also taken part in one or more of the collective creation projects on family violence, alcoholism, gun safety, AIDS, and suicide prevention that his classes had done in previous years. The students were already familiar with issues-based or applied approaches to drama. I introduced adaptations of Boal's *Theatre of the Oppressed* as an alternative dramatic form

The project was intended as a unit on Popular Theatre for the drama classes and a Popular Theatre project with a community of students. It was a participatory, performative inquiry into the experiences of these youth both for their own personal and social development and for the purposes of my research. The students' familiarity with improvisational drama and, more important, their comfort and willingness to use drama as a medium of expression and their openness to exploring issues through drama greatly assisted our process. I took on the roles of teacher, Popular Theatre facilitator, and coresearcher.

I engaged the students in a Popular Theatre process that drew on their experiences to examine issues they identified as relevant. The process began with a series of games and activities for group-building, trust-building, and skill development; moved on to the exploration of themes through brainstorming, image work, and discussion; and then into devising, storytelling of incidents from their lives, and the creation of scenes based on these stories. As we created the scenes, we animated them to explore the issues raised, using techniques adapted from Boal's *Theatre of the Oppressed*.

Our theme, "Life in the Sticks," emerged from the drama activities and discussion. Students felt that the issues they faced were determined by their rural environment. As one student put it, "It's because we've got nothing better to do. Kids get into all kinds of trouble because they are bored." Students brainstormed words and phrases in a Graffiti Wall activity and sculpted images of "Life in the Sticks." Students told stories about incidents from their lives, took on roles, and acted out situations based on the stories told, always looking for alternative responses. The process of devising and animating scenes allowed an in-depth, embodied discussion of students' perspectives regarding issues that affected their lives. The scenes we created, based on their stories and/or issues that arose during our exploration were about boredom, rule-breaking at school and its consequences, substance use, addiction, risky sex, gossip, gender relations, and interpersonal conflict. The drama raised questions inciting students to examine the issues and their beliefs and to reevaluate aspects of their lived experiences.

Toward the end of the process, I conducted an informal interview with a small group of students who volunteered to participate. I asked them what they thought the scenes we created were all about. Did they believe that the behavior depicted was determined by their rural environment? Ultimately, the students denied being victims of their environment; they rejected the notion of "at risk," claiming instead that their risky behavior was a matter of personal choice and habit. As one student said, "You drink just because you want to and do anything else because you want to." The notion of personal choice gave them back a sense of agency in and responsibility for their own behavior. This attitude had the potential to be empowering—a step toward finding solutions. Our work left me wondering, however, what motivated their risky choices.

The community action that was the culmination of our Popular Theatre project was a pair of performances/workshops of the scenes we had created, one for students at their school and another at a school in a neighboring town. We used a Forum Theatre model (Boal, 1974/1979) to engage audiences in further discussion of issues, searching for solutions or alternative responses to the "problems" presented.

Performative Re-Presentations

Following the Popular Theatre work with the students, my interpretation of "Life in the Sticks" began with a process of recursive writing. To talk about the Popular Theatre process, I needed to describe instances of our performance. I found an appropriate way of doing this through writing a series of scripted descriptions or "ethnodramatic" vignettes, 16 in all, depicting salient moments of our work together (Conrad, 2002; Saldaña, 2003). Based on the audio- and videotapes we made throughout the process, my journal and field notes, and students' journals, the scripts depict instances of performative interaction, discussion, the devising process, the scenes that students created, the animation of these scenes, responses to our performances, and the interviews I conducted with students.

My notes and transcriptions served as memory aides, but the scripts are also partly fictionalized (Banks & Banks, 1998) for ethical, thematic, and practical/writerly purposes. While the details do not always represent precisely what happened, to the extent to which it is possible, acknowledging that all interpretive work is inherently subjective (Clandinin & Connelly, 1994), I have tried to remain true to the substance of our work, and tried to capture the spirit of the interactions the scripted descriptions depict. For example, the scenes that students created were never formally scripted, but improvised anew each time they were performed, based on some cursory notes. My scripted recreations of these scenes are compilations based on videotapes of specific performances interwoven with details from other performances of the same scene and discussion that arose on various occasions as recorded in my field notes. As in any case, no text can claim to be free of the author's subjectivity (Banks & Banks, 1998); my scripts are constructions, but self-consciously so. I acknowledge that even in my choice of moments to script an interpretive process was involved, and thus my account of our participatory work is inherently partial.

The scripts are meant to be expressive and evocative rather than just explanatory. They are performative texts that bring the processes of academic interpretation and representation in closer touch with the actual performative events. My series of scripted vignettes describes the process involved in our Popular Theatre project in a way that preserves some of its performative quality. They embody the context and dynamics of the situations and preserve some of the authenticity of participants' voices and gestures. The scripts served as an initial level of interpretation for my subsequent interpretation/inquiry.

I offer here an excerpt from one of the vignettes I wrote as an example of the Popular Theatre process in action an improvised performance and the animation process that followed. I chose this moment to share because of the intriguing queries it raised. One of the scenes that students created, which we called "The Bus Trip," was based on an incident that occurred at the school the previous year, involving many of my students. It depicted a group of students illicitly drinking alcohol on the bus ride home from a class trip. In devising the scene, students took on the roles of characters and improvised the situation. The excerpt below shows a moment we enacted between two young men whose idea it was to buy the alcohol. This was an out-scene (a common Popular Theatre technique), a behind-the-scenes look at the original scene we created about the bus trip incident. In the midst of our reenactment, in the role as facilitator or Joker (Boal, 1974/1979), I stopped the action temporarily to question the actors in character (another Popular Theatre animation technique), to delve deeper into the moment of decision making and the motivation underlying their choice. All of the names in the vignette are code names that students gave themselves, a measure taken to protect their anonymity.

> *(The bus stops at the rest stop and they all get off. Shadzz and Daryl meet on the sidewalk.)*
>
> SHADZZ: *(to Daryl in character)* So give me some money, man.
>
> DARYL: What for?
>
> SHADZZ: I'm gonna get the stuff, remember?
>
> DARYL: Nah, forget it.
>
> SHADZZ: Come on, man, you said back there that you wanted to.
>
> DARYL: ... I don't know ...
>
> SHADZZ: Come on, it's just around the corner. I'll go get it and bring it back here.
>
> DARYL: Nah ...
>
> SHADZZ: What's the matter? Nobody's gonna know.
>
> DARYL: I don't know Shadzz.
>
> SHADZZ: Come on, Daryl.
>
> DARYL: Okay, what the hell ... here. *(Daryl gives Shadzz some money.)*
>
> TEACHER: *(Interrupting the improvisation.)* Stop it there for a minute. Daryl, I want to ask your character a question ... You hesitated to give him the money. Why?
>
> DARYL: I wasn't sure if I wanted to risk it.
>
> TEACHER: So, is there risk involved in what you're doing here?
>
> DARYL: Yeah.
>
> TEACHER: Go on.

DARYL: Well, we're kinda breaking the rules.

TEACHER: And where's the risk in that?

DARYL: Well, we might get caught.

SHADZZ: And expelled.

TEACHER: So there may be negative consequences to what you're doing ... Why do you do it?

DARYL: I don't know.

TEACHER: Shadzz, what about your character? *(Shadzz thinks about it.)*

SHADZZ: I don't know, just for the rush, I guess.

TEACHER: For the rush? Is that what risk-taking is about? Is that why someone might drink booze on a bus trip?

SHADZZ: Yeah, it's fun.

TEACHER: *(Addressing other students on stage and in the audience.)* Does doing something risky give you a rush?

(Echoes of agreement around the room.)

In the moment of Popular Theatre process depicted here, students enacted an incident based on their lived experiences, and with my intervention, explored the meaning behind their behavior revealing that they sometimes engaged in risky behavior "for the rush." In my further interpretation of our Popular Theatre work, I engaged in a discourse analysis (Fairclough, 1992) of "The Bus Trip" and other of my scripted descriptions to query students' responses to our work. The moments under analysis explored how students identified themselves, how they perceived their risky behavior, and their responses to the label "at risk."

Students' responses to my questions about risk-taking led me to further theoretical investigation of youth and risk. Elsewhere, I explore compelling theories on adolescent risk-taking (Lyng, 1993), theories on performative forms of resistance (Scott, 1990), and psychoanalytic interpretations of self-destructive behavior (Copjec, 1994) that provided further insight into risky youth behavior. An emergent realization that my interest in "at risk" was based on a desire to better understand my own risky experiences as a youth led to an autoethnographic inquiry (Conrad, 2003; Ellis & Bochner, 2000). The recovery of a collection of artifacts from my past (Slattery, 2001) and stories (Clandinin & Connelly, 2000) of my youthful risk-taking experiences resonated with what the students said and what theories revealed.

Conclusion

Combined, my interpretation of our Popular Theatre work, my theoretical investigations on youth and risk, and my autoethnographic understandings provide a layered exploration of youth behavior. This allowed me to reframe the concept of "at risk" (Roman, 1996) to include youths' perceptions of their behavior. A better understanding of youth and risk that more fully reflects their reality may better respond to their needs. Together, the Popular Theatre work with students, a participatory, performative approach to doing research, and my interpretation of it, present a counternarrative (Foucault, 1977) that interrupts the "common-sense" or taken-for-granted understandings of "at risk," providing a more complex picture than the one of deviance and deficiency currently suggested. My reinterpretation highlights youths' choice to engage in risky behavior, the enjoyment they gain from it, and its resistant quality—its potential to undermine unjust social structures. My study affirms the potential of Popular Theatre as a research method based on the new insight and critical understanding it has yielded (Denzin 1997; Lather, 1986) for my students and myself.

Notes

1. I find the label "at risk" extremely problematic. I am particularly disturbed by the way in which being an "at-risk" youth in Alberta highly correlates with being aboriginal (Alberta Learning, 2001). I explore the ethical implications of the label, the act of labeling, and the school and social structural factors that put youth "at risk" in my research. I problematize the fact that the majority of students at the school were of aboriginal descent while the teachers, myself included, were predominantly white.

2. Popular Theatre is the term I use to talk about a politically motivated type of participatory theater alternately referred to and/or closely allied to Boal's *Theatre of the Oppressed* (1974/1979); community theater (in Britain) or community-based performance; applied theater (Taylor, 2002); developmental theater in the developing world; some forms of documentary theater, collective creation, or sociodrama. Similar methods are employed in psychodrama or drama therapy contexts (Boal, 1995; Cohen-Cruz & Schutzman, 1994). Within drama/theater-in-education it is a form of issues-based, socially critical, or critically reflective drama (Errington, 1993).

3. Popular education is alternatively known as people's education or education for self-reliance (Africa), education for mass mobilization (Asia), cultural animation (Europe), and transformational education (North America). The Highlander Research and Education Center (*www.hrec.org*), a popular education and research organization in Tennessee, was established as early as 1932 and still sponsors educational programs and research into community prob-

lems. Catalyst Centre in Toronto (*www.catalystcentre.ca*) a nonprofit workers co-op, and the Centre for Popular Education, University of Technology, Sydney (*www.cpe.uts.edu.au*) promote popular education, research, and community development to advance positive social change.

4. While Popular Theatre takes various forms, Boal's *Theatre of the Oppressed* is perhaps one of the best known, with organizations around the world practicing adaptations of these techniques including the Center of the Theatre of the Oppressed in Rio and Paris (*www.ctrio.com.br*); FORMAAT in Holland (*www.formaat.org*); Pedagogy and Theatre of the Oppressed based at the University of Omaha (*www.unomaha.edu/~pto*); Theatre of the Oppressed Laboratory in New York (*www.toplab.org*); Mandala Center Seattle, Washington (*www.mandalaforchange.com*); Headlines Theatre in Vancouver (*www.headlinestheatre.com*); Rohd's (1998) Hope is Vital (HIV) program; New York University's Creative Arts Team (*www.nyu.edu/Gallatin/creativearts*); and the Centre for Applied Theatre Research in Australia (Taylor, 2002). Further approaches to *Theatre of the Oppressed* are described in Cohen-Cruz and Schutzman's (1994) *Playing Boal: Theatre, Therapy, Activism.* Other forms of Popular Theatre are explored in Prentki and Selman's (2000) *Popular Theatre in Political Culture: Britain and Canada in Focus.*

5. The Highlander Research and Education Center and the Society for Participatory Research in Asia (*www.pria.org*) are among the organizations that promote participatory research. Orlando Fals-Borda, a leading figure in the development of participatory research in Columbia, calls his line of research participatory action research. Participatory research also allies with socially critical action research (Tripp, 1990) and transformative research (Deshler & Selener, 1991).

6. In the past few years I have attended presentations at conferences and read about research using forms, including Readers' Theatre, poetry, photography, music, collage, drawing, sculpture, quilting, stained glass, performance, and dance. For examples, see Diamond and Mullen (1999) and recent special issues of journals dedicated to arts-based research including *Qualitative Inquiry, 9*(2); *Alberta Journal of Educational Research, 48*(3); *Journal of Curriculum Theorizing, 17*(2); and the Arts-based Approaches to Educational Research Special Interest Group of the American Educational Research Association (*www.usd.edu/aber*).

7. Mimesis, the human faculty for imitation or representation of reality, as it is put to use in Popular Theatre and performance ethnography, has ethical implications that I explore in relation to my research in detail elsewhere.

References

Alberta Learning. (2001). *Removing barriers to high school completion: Final report.* Retrieved October 22, 2003, from *www.learning.gov.ab.ca/k_12/special/ Barrier Report.pdf*

Austin, J. L. (1975). *How to do things with words.* Cambridge, MA: Harvard University Press.

Banks, A., & Banks, S. (1998). The struggle over facts and fictions. In A. Banks &

S. Banks (Eds.), *Fiction and social research: By ice or fire* (pp. 11–29). London: AltaMira Press.

Boal, A. (1979). *Theatre of the oppressed* (C. McBride & M. McBride, Trans.). London: Pluto Press. (Original work published 1974)

Boal, A. (1995). *The rainbow of desire* (A. Jackson, Trans.). London: Routledge.

Boal, A. (1999). *Legislative theatre: Using performance to make politics* (A. Jackson, Trans.). London: Routledge.

Brecht, B. (1964). *Brecht on theater* (J. Willett, Trans.). New York: Hill & Wang. (Original work published 1957)

Butler, J. P. (1997). *Excitable speech: A politics of the performance.* New York: Routledge.

Clandinin, J., & Connelly, M. (1994). Personal experience methods. In N. Denzin & Y. Lincoln (Eds.), *Handbook of qualitative research* (pp. 413–427). Thousand Oaks, CA: Sage.

Clandinin, J., & Connelly, M. (2000). *Narrative inquiry: Experience and story in qualitative research.* San Francisco: Jossey-Bass.

Cohen-Cruz, J., & Schutzman, M. (Eds.). (1994). *Playing Boal: Theatre, therapy, activism.* London: Routledge.

Conquergood, D. (1985). Performing as a moral act: Ethical dimensions of the ethnography of performance. *Literature in Performance, 5*(2), 1–13.

Conquergood, D. (1998). Beyond the text: Toward a performative cultural politics. In S. Dailey (Ed.), *The future of performance studies: Visions and revisions* (pp. 25–36). Annandale, VA: National Communication Association.

Conrad, D. (2002). Drama as arts-based pedagogy and research: Media advertising and inner-city youth. *Alberta Journal of Educational Research, 48*(3), 254–268.

Conrad, D. (2003). Unearthing personal history: Autoethnography and artifacts inform research on youth risk-taking. *Journal of Social Theory in Art Education, 23,* 44–58.

Copjec, J. (1994). *Read my desire: Lacan against the historicists.* Cambridge, MA: MIT Press.

Courtney, R. (1988). Columbus here and now. In D. Booth & A. Martin-Smith (Eds.), *Recognizing Richard Courtney: Selected writings on drama and education* (pp. 55–61). Markham, ON, Canada: Pembroke.

Denzin, N. K. (1997). *Interpretive ethnography: Ethnographic practices for the 21st century.* London: Sage.

Denzin, N. K. (2003). *Performance ethnography: Critical pedagogy and the politics of culture.* Thousand Oaks, CA: Sage.

Deshler, D., & Selener, D. (1991). Transformative research: In search of a definition. *Convergence, 24*(3), 9–22.

Diamond, C., & Mullen, C. (1999). *The postmodern educator: Arts-based inquiries and teacher development.* New York: Peter Lang.

Eisner, E. (1997). The promise and perils of alternative forms of data representation. *Educational Researcher, 26*(6), 4–10.

Ellis, C., & Bochner, A. (2000). Autoethnography, personal narrative, reflexivity: Researcher as subject. In N. K. Denzin & Y. S. Lincoln, (Eds.), *The handbook of qualitative research* (pp. 733–768). Thousand Oaks, CA: Sage.

Errington, E. (1993). Orientations toward drama education in the nineties. In E.

Errington (Ed.), *Arts education: Beliefs, practices and possibilities* (pp.183–192). Geelong, Australia: Deakin University Press.

Fabian, J. (1990). *Power and performance: Ethnographic explorations through proverbial wisdom and theatre in Shaba, Zaire.* Madison: University of Wisconsin Press.

Fairclough, N. (1992). *Discourse and social change.* Cambridge, MA: Polity Press.

Fals-Borda, O., & Rahman, M. (Eds.). (1991). *Action and knowledge: Breaking the monopoly with participatory action-research.* New York: Apex Press.

Finley, S. (2003). Arts-based inquiry in QI: Seven years from crisis to guerrilla warfare. *Qualitative Inquiry, 9*(2), 281–296.

Foucault, M. (1977). *Language, counter-memory, practice: Selected essays and interviews*(D. Bouchard & S. Simon, Trans.). Ithaca, NY: Cornell University Press.

Freire, P. (1970). *Pedagogy of the oppressed* (M. B. Ramos, Trans.). New York: Continuum.

Freire, P. (1988). Creating alternative research methods: Learning to do it by doing it. In S. Kemmis & R. McTaggart (Eds.), *The action research reader* (pp. 291–313). Geelong, Australia: Deakin University Press.

Garoian, C. (1999). *Performing pedagogy: Toward an art of politics.* Albany: State University of New York Press.

Kidd, R. (1982). *The popular performing arts, nonformal education and social change in the Third World: A bibliography and review essay.* Toronto, ON: Centre for the study of education in developing countries.

Kidd, R., & Byram, M. (1978). Popular theatre: Technique for participatory research. *Participatory Research Project* (Working Paper No. 5). Toronto.

Lather, P. (1986). Issues of validity in openly ideological research: Between a rock and a soft place. *Interchange, 17*(4), 63–84.

Lyng, S. (1993). Dysfunctional risk taking: Criminal behavior as edgework. In N. Bell & R. Bell (Eds.), *Adolescent risk taking* (pp. 107–130). Newbury Park, CA: Sage.

McTaggart, R. (Ed.). (1997). *Participatory action research: International contexts and consequences.* Albany: State University of New York Press.

National Coalition of Advocates for Students. (1985). *Barriers to excellence: Our children "at-risk."* Boston: Author.

Norris, J. (2000). Drama as research: Realizing the potential of drama in education as a research methodology. *Youth Theatre Journal, 14,* 40–51.

Park, P., Brydon-Miller, M., Hall, B., & Jackson, T. (Eds.). (1993). *Voices of change: Participatory research in the United States and Canada.* Westport, CT: Bergin & Garvey.

Prentki, T., & Selman, J. (2000). *Popular theatre in political culture: Britain and Canada in focus.* Portland, OR: Intellect Books.

Rohd, M. (1998). *Theatre for community, conflict and dialogue: The Hope is Vital training manual.* Portsmouth, NH: Heinemann.

Roman, L. (1996). Spectacle in the dark: Youth as transgression, display, and repression. *Educational Theory, 46*(1), 1–22.

Salazar, M. (1991). Young laborers in Bogotá: Breaking authoritarian ramparts. In O. Fals-Borda & M. Rahman (Eds.), *Action and knowledge: Breaking the monopoly with participatory action-research* (pp. 54–63). New York: Apex Press.

Saldaña, J. (1999). Playwriting with data: Ethnographic performance texts. *Youth Theatre Journal, 13,* 60–71.

Saldaña, J. (2003). Dramatizing data: A primer. *Qualitative Inquiry, 9*(2), 218–236.

Scott, J. (1990). *Domination and the arts of resistance: Hidden transcripts.* New Haven, CT: Yale University Press.

Schechner, R. (1985). *Between theater and anthropology.* Philadelphia: University of Pennsylvania Press.

Slattery, P. (2001). The educational researcher as artist working within. *Qualitative Inquiry, 7*(4), 370–398.

Taylor, P. (2002). The applied theatre: Building stronger communities. *Youth Theatre Journal, 16,* 88–95.

Taussig, M. (1993). *Mimesis and alterity: A particular history of the senses.* New York: Routledge.

Tripp, D. (1990). Socially critical action research. *Theory into Practice, 29*(3), 158–166.

Turner, V. (1986). *The anthropology of performance.* New York: PAJ.

CHAPTER 6

~~~~~

Dance and Movement

Dance becomes this place of dynamic possibility where the invisible and visible become partners.

—CELESTE N. SNOWBER (2002, p. 22)

Famed photographer Annie Leibovitz recently commented that after many efforts at photographing dance she realized it was an impossible goal, for, as she put it, "dance is in the air, it's just in the air." As dance belongs entirely to the moment, existing only in performance (and performances are never entirely identical), it is difficult to pin down for descriptive purposes. Elaine Clark-Rapley asserts that dance "exemplifies the doing side of living" (1999, p. 89) and is best described with action words.

Despite the dynamic nature of dance, ritual and discipline shape both the many uses of dance as well as the dancer's body, a highly disciplined instrument (and the focus of earlier scholarship on dance and gender). Furthermore, the abstract character of dance is also linked to its reconstituting of many other art forms. In fact, dance combines elements of all the other art forms in this book: it is musical, performative, visual, poetic, autobiographical, and can serve narrative. Of course, although it draws on these other arts, dance cannot be reduced to any of them nor be their sum total. Although it is an abstract art form, and perhaps because of it, dance has been referred to as a "universal language," the "mother of all tongues," and the "mirror of the soul" (Warren, 1993). Nevertheless, as reviewed with respect to music in Chapter 4, dance too is historically and culturally bound and thus differs within and across contexts.

Dance is in many ways the most abstract art form explored in this book. As reviewed in Chapter 5, performance studies are far more com-

179

mon than the methodological uses of dance; however, dance is also a *genre of performance* and thus techniques that have emerged and been refined in performance-based methods may be useful as dance-based methods emerge. Although traditional performance-based methods such as ethnodrama may have a more obvious link to data representation (e.g., via scripting), and dance by contrast is viewed as more abstract, commonalities remain. Both mediums can be used to create empathetic connection, raise awareness, educate, promote social justice, and are embodied forms of presentation (when performed).

Dance can incorporate words as well and can even be based on a script, which may or may not be summarized for audiences in written form (as is the case when ballets such as "Romeo and Juliet," "Swan Lake," and many others are performed). In other words, dance can communicate narratives, although unconventionally. I suggest that researchers presenting their data via dance consider an accompanying textual component of representation in order to contextualize the performance, just as many visual artists include statements with their work.

There is emergent theoretical scholarship that explores dance within the context of Marxist views, positing that dance transcends historical time. Clark-Rapley (1999) argues that Karl Marx's analysis of human activity centers on instrumental human action, with purposive material ends. She suggests that dance is a form of transformative human action that expresses an individual's being *without purposive ends* and can thus support communal relations (as opposed to alienated relations) and aid, not diminish, self-actualization. Moreover, improvisational dance breaks patterned movements and promotes discovery, differing greatly from Marx's view of labor and social control. Clark-Rapley conducted ethnographic research in a university dance class with 24 undergraduates. Her participant observation research included field notes, audiotaping, videotaping, and dancers' journals. From this data she made several observations about dance improvisation from an outsider's vantage point. Clark-Rapley writes:

> Improvising activity is distinct from practical activity since it begins and ends with a unified relation between the dancer (as "subject") and the dance (as "object"). The relation of the dancer to the dance, and of the dancer to the dance process, is a relation of unity that blurs the subject/object distinction: the dancer is the activity and the dancer is the dance. (p. 92)

In part what this research suggests is that dance has a *transcendent, consciousness-raising potential*—a theme that reemerges throughout dance scholarship.

The transcendent and consciousness-raising capacities of dance can be harnessed by qualitative researchers to build methods practices congruent with related research purposes. For example, social action researchers may use dance performances to celebrate differences and/or transcend social and economic barriers. Researchers working from queer studies, feminist, or multicultural perspectives might consider dance as a representational vehicle for its capacity to foster consciousness-raising. In this regard, research participants might be asked to engage in creative movement exercises in addition to in-depth or focus-group interviews as a source of consciousness-raising and reflection during data analysis. This is addressed in the section, later in this chapter, on multimethod research that focuses on the use of creative movement in a project about consciousness-raising.

Despite only recently being explored as a method of inquiry across multiple disciplines, dance has been a subject of anthropological studies of folklore and folk life for many decades (as well as dance education). In a special issue of the *Australian Journal of Anthropology* (December 2000), on the anthropology of dance, Rosita Henry reviews the new directions being chartered in anthropological studies of dance. She posits that there has been a great surge in anthropological studies of dance and movement in the past two decades (formerly a marginal topic of inquiry). She suggests the increase in "dance studies" results from new understandings about how dance is a dynamic, productive force in social life. On behalf of the contributors in the special issue Henry writes:

> We theorise dance practices as domains of lived experience, and position movement as a performative moment of social interchange that is not merely reflective of prior political, personal, social and cosmological relations, but also constitutive of the relationship of them. We argue that a renegotiation of the relationship between dance and anthropology is required so that dance is given full recognition as an active, fraught and dynamic force in human social life ... we contest conventional boundaries of dance concepts by taking as our focus of study a dialectical space of performative action where discursive political, aesthetic, ritual and cultural forms are produced. Attention to the ways in which movement is able to infuse space with socio-religious and socio-political meaning requires that dance practices be viewed as historically embodied, contextual, discursive and interconnected domains of lived experience. (2000, p. 1)

In her article "Reprise: On Dance Ethnography" Deidre Sklar (2000) reflects on how when her essay "On Dance Ethnography" was published in 1991 there was very little literature on the subject, but a decade later dance and movement scholarship had blossomed, creating a range of theories, methods, and case studies executed within the categories of "cultural studies in dance," "performance studies," "anthropology of dance," "anthropology of human movement," "dance ethnology," and "ethnochoreology."

Arguably, the low status dance has historically received in academic research mirrors the low status dance enjoys relative to other arts (as evidenced in many ways, including the pay scale for dancers as compared with other artists at a comparable career stage). Stinson (1995, 1998, 2004) explains how the low status of dance is inextricably linked to its association with women and women's bodies. Nevertheless, the exploration of dance in cultural (and expressive) anthropology reflects the centrality of dance and movement to many cultural rituals as well as its productive role in culture. Dance therefore can produce insights into various aspects of different cultures.

In this vein, Caroline Joan Picart (2002) studied American ballroom dance in order to learn about the gendered nature of interaction expressed in this style of dance. Picart's research provides many insights into the gendered politics of leading/following, how feminine and masculine bodies are produced, and issues pertaining to the "gaze."

The recent increase in dance as a methodological tool results from the overall increase in performance studies (explored in Chapter 5), the surge in embodiment research, rises in phenomenology, and increases in health and education research that have identified dance as a therapeutic tool and vehicle for building positive social characteristics (which is now being applied to arts-based research practices).

Within the context of increases in performance and dance studies, *movement analysis* has emerged as an important research method that can enhance the practice of traditional qualitative methods such as ethnography and interview by helping researchers systematically attend to all of the gestured and other nonverbal communication that occurs within qualitative research (see Daly, 1988). In addition, as qualitative researchers started seriously working with other art forms, so too have they incorporated dance into methodological practices.

- How do social researchers incorporate the body into their work? How have advances in embodiment research contributed to the use of dance in social research?

- How are phenomenologists advancing our understanding of all experience as bodily in ways that promote the body as a central source of data or representational vehicle?

Embodiment Research and Phenomenology

Dance cannot be understood without attention to the fact that it is necessarily an embodied art form. Early 20th-century choreographer Ted Shawn proclaimed: "Dance is the only art of which we ourselves are the stuff of which it is made." Over the past several decades "the body" has garnered considerable attention in academic scholarship largely due to the advances of feminist, postmodern, poststructural, and psychoanalytic theories of embodiment. Although this is a broad range of theoretical traditions, what these critical perspectives have in common is attention to social power and a position that claims all social actors to be *embodied* actors, and thus experience is necessarily embodied. Social reality is experienced from embodied standpoints. Of interest to many social justice–oriented researchers working within these traditions are the ways in which bodies become raced, sexed, and gendered.

Renowned scholar Elizabeth Grosz (1994) distinguishes "inscriptive" and "the lived body" approaches to embodiment research. The inscribed body serves as a site where social meanings are created and resisted. Influenced by the work of Michel Foucault (1976) and Susan Bordo (1989), Grosz writes, "The body is not outside of history, for it is produced through and in history" (1994, p. 148). The inscriptions may be "subtle" or "violent" but are ultimately cumulative in effect (p. 141). The way we sex or gender or race the body is deeply implicated in existing relations of power (pp. 141–142).

It is in theories of "the lived body" that a clear link between embodiment research and phenomenology is evidenced. In embodiment scholarship "the lived body" refers to people's experiential knowledge. Grosz is influenced by Merleau-Ponty (1962), who posited that we must look at the "necessary interconnectedness" of the mind and body (Grosz, 1994, p. 86). Merleau-Ponty argued that experience exists between the mind and body. Therefore, the body is not viewed as an object but rather as the "condition and context" through which social actors have relations to objects and through which they give and receive information (Grosz, 1994, p 86). Put simply, the body is a tool through which meaning is created. Tami Spry (2006), an innovative qualitative researcher, suggests that in order to access experiential knowledge researchers must find ways to access "enfleshed knowledge." This is a holistic view of experience as embodied and of the mind and body as interconnected. These advances in our understanding of embodiment and the physicality of experience, which have largely emerged in theoretical scholarship, serve as a part of the context for various methodological innovations, including recent explorations of dance and movement as methodological tools.

For example, Stinson (2004) explains that dance teaches a person to feel from the inside, and correspondingly how to use the body as a source of knowledge and locus of meaning (p. 163). Drawing on theories of embodiment as she reflects on dance and movement as legitimate methods of inquiry, Stinson proposes that the body is a microcosm of the world and a venue for understanding its meaning (p. 160). Moreover, influenced by phenomenological approaches to knowledge-building, she further suggests that the entire body can be viewed as an experiential and memory repository for what we "know," which may emerge through dance in unexpected ways (p. 160).

An extension of this theoretical and methodological work is in the area of health care. The body, as well as the mind–body connection, have long been a part of empirical health research and alternative health-care practices.

- How do health-care researchers and practitioners employ dance as a therapeutic tool? What do these practices say about the arts, the public–private dichotomy, and the relationship between the mind and body?

- How is dance used in education research to foster dimensions of positive self-concept?

Health and Education Research: Dance as a Therapeutic Tool

In recent decades there has been a significant surge in health researchers and practitioners, as well as others, who are (re)exploring the mental, psychological, and physical health benefits of dance and movement. It is almost as if researchers *rediscovered* these arts-based therapeutic tools (in the age of globalization), long employed by various indigenous groups as well as a part of standard care in many Eastern health care and lifestyle practices. For example, Yvette Kim (2004) writes about the positive benefits of ancient "multidimensional healing" practices. Her work focuses on a teaching workshop where indigenous methods of healing are used, including dance and music. Some researchers working at the cutting edge of this field, such as Ebru Yaman (2003), refer to arts-based therapies like dance and music as "expressive therapies" that can be both *healing* and *validating*—a combination of outcomes that explains why the benefits of arts-based therapies are of interest to practitioners in both health care and education. With respect to the latter, Fay Burstin (2004) proposes that movement and music can be used in education to help develop communication and literacy skills. Bernie Warren (1993) posits dance as an alternative creative outlet for shy people.[1] Jennifer Kingma

(2004) conducted research that explores the link between dance and markers of positive self-esteem such as confidence.[2]

- In what ways are sociologists and anthropologists employing dance in their research?
- What methodological possibilities exist at the intersection of dance and social inquiry?
- How is rigor achieved in these experimental designs?

Dance as a Methodological Innovation

Social and behavioral scientists include dance in their scholarly research in numerous ways. Although anthropologists have long studied dance as a source of cultural information (a *subject* of inquiry), it is only in the past couple of decades that a broader range of qualitative researchers have begun to incorporate dance into their research, not just as a subject of inquiry (although this is important), but also as a *methodological device.*

Dance can facilitate social research in two primary ways. First, dance can serve as a source of data and consequently as a *data collection method* (or part of a data collection procedure). Second, dance can serve as a *representational form,* a methodological innovation that is only recently being explored by qualitative researchers. The purpose of these methods is typically *discovery*—a way of adding depth to our understanding of a particular subject.

One general area where dance has considerable but largely untapped potential to contribute to our understanding is in regards to the public–private dialectic. Dance as a discipline merges the public and private, or inner and outer worlds if we are to adopt the discourse of dance education, because the dancer's body is always moving within an environment. Therefore, as these cutting-edge research practices are used and refined, it is likely that we will see more scholarship (outside of dance education) that explores this relationship. In addition, despite the abstract "nonscience" nature of art (or perhaps as a response to it), some of the dance-based methods proposed by social researchers are among the most systematic offered in the burgeoning field of arts-based research practices.

Dance and Data Collection

As mentioned earlier, dance as a part of data collection occurs on a continuum where dance can serve variously as a source of information or a method of data collection. Beginning with the former, anthropologists (and more recently sociologists) have examined dance in many different cultural and cross-cultural contexts as a part of normative cultural practices, religious customs, celebratory rituals, and many other cultural rituals. Sklar identifies this as the "sociopolitical trajectory," one of two major ways contemporary anthropologists employ dance and movement into their methodology (2000, p. 70). Dance research can also be a means for gaining insight into the cultural construction of gender (and similar issues).

Diane C. Freedman (1991) studied Romanian dance couples to learn about courtship and marriage rituals that center on dance in a particular village. More generally, the research project used dance as a means to explore gender relations in this environment. Freedman's research centers on dance as a *subject of inquiry* and not a methodological tool—the former of which is not the focus of this chapter. However, her systematic approach to analyzing dance may be of great value to researchers starting to work with dance as a research tool and attempting to develop rigorous protocols.

Freedman designed a research project using the rigorous *Laban movement analysis* (LMA) method that systematically studies movement. This method developed out of dance methodology and the second major research trajectory: *kinesthetic,* which investigates movement itself as a way of knowing (Sklar, 2000, p. 70). LMA employs "effort/shape" approaches to the analysis of dance and movement. According to Freedman, the approach considers three perspectives: (1) use of the body, (2) use of the space, and (3) use of effort. Additional factors for LMA include which body parts, how they move in space, and the type of energy that motivates the movement (Freedman, 1991). The body and the space are also further categorized. Dimensions of the body include height, weight, and depth. The three axes of space are horizontal, vertical, and sagittal (front to back). With these factors in mind, Freedman designed a systematic strategy for analyzing the Romanian dance couples in her study.

First, she spent 20 hours watching a tape of a 2-hour dance. She also looked at other dances and gathered additional relevant information from other villages. Based on this initial data-collection phase, Freedman created a list of "effort/shape" factors and determined that her unit of analysis in the next data-collection phase would be 5-second intervals of the dance. In addition to developing a coding procedure in this inductive format (similar to some grounded theory approaches to data collection and simultaneous analysis and assessment) she also used these data to create a "cultural profile" consisting of characteristics shared by the villagers. A component of this profile was a list of dissimilar characteristics that Freedman then further analyzed in search of emergent patterns, such as a gendered division. In fact, there were significant gender-related differences that offered insights into cultural notions of gender, courtship, and marriage. Freedman notes: "Movement differences between men and women are part of the meaningful sign system by which gender is defined. In the dance code, certain movement signs are selected which emphasize gender differences" (p. 344). In this study, Freedman concluded that dance movements are central to mate selection and that such movements are profoundly gendered.

Although Freedman's study centers primarily on dance as data and not as a methodological practice, how can the techniques employed in her study serve methodological innovation? For example, research participants asked to engage in creative movement during data collection, a practice that may result in a video recording of the experience, could be analyzed with the LMA method. The various factors for analysis (body parts, use of space, etc.) could be developed in accord with the particular project (which may center on individual experience or relationships between participants). Another example where this method could be adapted by social researchers focuses on the representation stage of research. Many performance-based methods include pre- and postperformance components. Audiences gathered to view a research-based dance performance could be given analysis sheets created by the researcher(s). These sheets, which could also serve as data, could be constructed based on the LMA strategy, covering the dimensions pertinent to a particular project.

Dance can also serve as a data-collection method in comparative research. Beck, Martinez, and Lires (1999) used dance in their empirical study about interpretive skills in multicultural and multimedia contexts. Speaking to the broad and rigorous ways in which dance can serve methodology, their study incorporated dance into an experiment research design. The overall goal of the study was to determine what interactive media or dance experiences most assist people with their interpretive skills. During the preliminary phase of the research project the researchers had two experts, one dance historian and one composer of dance music, interpret an Aztec dance called the Concheros dance. The researchers observed how the two experts interpreted the dance. Based on these observations Beck and colleagues developed a list of four interpretive skills they would later use as benchmarks on which to test research participants. For this project 60 female student teachers enrolled in a course on "art and music teaching methods" were divided into two groups—one control group and one experimental group. Both groups were taught the Concheros dance and made headdresses similar to those worn by the Aztecs, which they wore during the dance. One week later the experimental group watched a video performance and engaged with a 90-minute interactive CD-ROM. Then, both groups wrote interpretive essays about how the dance reflects the society and what different parts of the dance express. The experimental group scored higher on the test.

Although this study presents one interesting methodological use of dance, an altered research design may be helpful to consider as well. As it was carried out, their research ultimately only considers the added value of the video and CD-ROM. Another way of conducting this research would have been to have one group learn how to perform the dance (by dancing themselves) while wearing the traditional costumes they made. The other group would learn about the dance only by watching the video and then engaging with the interactive CD-ROM. The two groups would then write the interpretive essay. Within this alternate design strategy, the essay scores would ultimately compare the effectiveness of the *first-hand experience* of the dance with the *removed multimedia experience* of the video viewing and computer-based engagement. This kind of project could add considerably to our understanding of experiential versus media-based educational practices.

The final data-collection procedures explored in this chapter are "improvisational dance" and "body narratives." Celeste Snowber (2002) writes about dance as a method for garnering knowledge. She is specifically interested in investigating the connection between autobiographical narrative and dance. Snowber claims that *improvisational dance* acknowledges and calls on multiplicity—the multiple lives one has, the multiple dimensions of self, and multiple meanings. Therefore, improvisational dance as a research method can provide insights into the life of the performer and create a space for dialogue. As with other methodological uses of dance, improvisational dance as a method of inquiry merges multiple ways of knowing. Snowber explains that the practice uses "phenomenological curriculum research, narrative inquiry, autobiographical writing, and performative inquiry" (p. 20). Moreover, dance allows a relationship to develop between the outer world and our bodies, as also noted by education researchers who use dance for esteem-building. Our bodies experience things first via our physical interaction with the world; therefore, there are kinds of data that our bodies experience before our minds (Snowber, 2002). From this position Snowber argues that dance is an expression of our bodies and bodily knowledge and is therefore a valid method for exploring and representing data.

Snowber suggests an additional dance-based method, termed *body narratives*, that combines dance and autobiographical narratives. Body narratives are therefore a methodological option for researchers who want to explore the possibilities of a dance-based method while also retaining the tool of narrative (and "the word," more broadly). This method may also suggest a way to create and represent autoethnographic research (itself on the rise, as discussed in Chapter 2). The primary purpose of this practice is *discovery*. Snowber writes, "I would suggest that the process of improvisation and creation in all the arts is an embodied ritual which leads us into not-knowing, and ultimately into knowing" (2002, p. 28). Furthermore, aspects of the invisible, or that which may not be actively remembered in the conscious mind, may emerge through dance.

Dance, Data Collection, and Multimethod Research

Dance or movement can be employed as one of several data collection tools in a multimethod research design. As with all multimethod research, the point isn't simply to "add" methods but rather to let them inform each other (Hesse-Biber & Leavy, 2005).

Carol Picard (2000) provides an example of how dance can be incorporated into health-care research as one of multiple methods. Picard's study examines the process by which women at midlife expand their consciousness via two different means of expression: narrative and creative movement. Her sample consisted of 17 women at midlife and her data collection occurred in three phases: first an in-depth interview, then a creative movement group, and third a follow-up in-depth interview (all of which occurred within a 5-week period for each woman).

The first interview lasted 50 minutes to 2 hours, 75 minutes on average. In this interview the women were asked to share what was most meaningful in their lives. The second phase, the creative movement component, occurred in the context of the group (the women were divided into two groups and were allotted 3½ hours for the group session). None of the women had participated in a creative movement group before, so it was a new experience. Each group began with a series of trust exercises so that the women would feel comfortable moving their bodies within the group. Then each woman was given an opportunity to express, via movement, what was most meaningful to her. She then had an opportunity to describe what the movement meant to her, and then to repeat her movement. Finally, there was a group-closure exercise followed by a breathing exercise. The creative movement sessions were videotaped and analyzed by the researcher for "meaning and overall movement qualities, such as the overall use of space, and the complexity, length, or brevity of the whole of the expression" (p. 152). The verbal data from the videotapes was transcribed and also analyzed. The researcher then created a diagram of each participant's patterns (adding a visual component to the interpretive process). In the second interview session the diagram was presented to the participant, who was given an opportunity to revise it. Next, each woman viewed the videotape of her movement with the researcher and was asked to reflect on the videotape as well as the entire research process.

In this study, the different methods all "speak to each other" and are a part of an *integrated approach* to knowledge-building. In other words, the methods operate synergistically. The traditional qualitative interview component and creative movement component are related, both seeking to yield insights about the same thing: what is most meaningful in the participant's life. The latter interview then provided a reflective, collaborative opportunity for the participant to clarify the meaning derived from the data as well as to reflect on what the experience has been like for her. Picard reports that the women reflected the experience promoted "self-discovery" and that the group component made the women feel valued and accepted by others. Moreover, all but one of the women reported that the creative movement they viewed on the videotape accurately reflected their narrative (in the anomalous experience important data were garnered, as the participant noted a disjuncture between her life as it was and as she imagined it, reflected in her narrative versus creative movement expressions).

For many of the women, the combination of verbally sharing their narrative and then creatively using their bodies in a public space provided an opportunity to reflect on their lives that extended beyond the confines of the research project. One participant even reported using creative movement at home after participating in the study. Picard concludes that the use of creative movement added to her research on how women's consciousness develops and that the participants themselves validated the use of this form of expression. Finally, she proposes that the use of multiple methods of expression can add depth and dimension to social research.

- How can dance be used as a performance-based method of representation?
- What issues arise when translating traditional qualitative data into a choreographed dance? Specifically, what are the potential advantages and disadvantages of the abstract nature of dance with respect to generating meaning(s)?
- What strategies are available for garnering trustworthiness and validity?

Dance as a Representational Form

Although it is a relatively underutilized practice in social research, some qualitative researchers have begun to explore dance as a form of data representation. This innovation is an outgrowth of a move toward alternative representational forms, the inevitable exploration of embodiment theoretical scholarship with respect to methodology and representation, and the overall increase in performance studies and particularly performance as a representational form as reviewed in the last chapter. The single largest contribution to scholarship on dance as a representational form is the volume *Dancing the Data*, edited by Carl Bagley and Mary Beth Cancienne (2002). In this text, Donald Blumenfeld-Jones (2002) explores the art–research connection that emerges when dance is used as a medium for representation.

Blumenfeld-Jones (2002) offers several observations and suggestions for how to conceptualize the dance-representation possibility and how to most effectively realize its potential. In this regard, he suggests that dance can be used to *convey meaning*—meaning as intended by the researcher. However, congruent with larger issues pertaining to art and social inquiry, he notes that art necessarily invites several interpretations at once. This does not mean that all interpretations are accurate (a concern that guides much of the criticism of qualitative research—a fear of everything being relative and all-inclusive). With all of this in mind, Blumenfeld-Jones argues that when working with dance as a representational vehicle, researchers must be very careful to use movements that convey only a range of meanings that are appropriate to the theme of which he or she is communicating dimensions. To most effectively enact this advice, I would also suggest an external review phase of research. Specifically, after the choreography has been created the research design could allow for a "pilot performance" for a sample of colleagues or experts who could provide the researcher with feedback regarding their impressions, how they interpreted the various movements, and what themes emerge from the dance. The researcher could then make modifications as necessary in order to evoke the limited set of interpretations he or she is after. Moreover, this design adds a dimension of validity to a new and highly experimental methodological practice that has not yet yielded a consistent criterion for assessing trustworthiness.

Carl Bagley and Mary Beth Cancienne's (2002) research provides an excellent empirical example of their attempts at using dance as a representational form in education research. Bagley is an education researcher and Cancienne is a choreographer, dance expert, and scholar. While attending a conference Cancienne was asked, with very little notice, to present a dance representing a dataset. Ultimately, the last-minute attempt failed; however, Cancienne wanted to try again under more optimal circumstances, convinced that dance as a representational form could contribute to social knowledge.

For the project they developed, Bagley collected the data on the topic "Impact of School Choice on Families Whose Children Had Special Educational Needs." He conducted interviews and then selected 10 of the interviews as the final dataset for the collaborative project, at which point Cancienne was given the data so that she could create a dance that she thought represented it. Cancienne constructed an interpretative dance with words in order to preserve parents' voices and best convey the data. She portrayed the voices in abstract ways (that were nonetheless clear in meaning). For example, at one point a dancer drew the name of a child on the floor with her foot when the parent spoke of the child being unable to write.

Bagley felt the project succeeded because people could connect with the data due to how it was represented. Moreover, the researchers viewed the data (or information) itself as the same as in traditional textual form, but the dance performance infused it with new light and insight. In this respect, they concluded that the dance added *new dimensions* rather than new understandings (2002, p. 15).

Finally, as with all art- and performance-based methods, the representation of the data in a dance format opened up a space for multiple meanings to emerge, although within the confines of a set of themes. Bagley and Cancienne write:

> In "dancing the data" we were able to facilitate a movement away from and disruption of the monovocal and monological nature of the voice in the print-based paper. Through a choreographed performance we were provided with an opportunity to encapture the multivocal and dialogical, as well as to cultivate multiple meanings, interpretations, and perspectives that might engage the audience in a recognition of textual diversity and complexity. (2002, p. 16)

In this vein, dance as a representational strategy has the potential to add both depth and texture to the insights created out of traditional qualitative practice.

Bagley and Cancienne's groundbreaking exploration of dance as a representational form can be viewed as an example of what is possible. What other kinds of interview or ethnographic data could be represented via dance? Interview data on a range of "feeling experiences" might be appropriate. Examples include grief, illness, depression, posttraumatic stress, love, powerlessness, and many other topics. Likewise, the personal experience associated with sexism, racism, or heterosexism may also be expressed via dance performance.

Checklist of Considerations

✓ How will the use of dance or movement enhance or enable my research objectives?

✓ When employing dance during data collection, what specific methodology will be implemented? What other methods or data-gathering techniques will be used in conjunction with dance? How do the methods inform each other?

✓ When using improvisational dance methods, how does the method converge with the theoretical framework, and how does it speak to the research objectives (i.e., discovery)?

✓ When using dance as a representational form, what am I "after"? How will I evaluate my success? What strategies for strengthening trustworthiness will be implemented?

Conclusion

The aim of this chapter has been to review the major uses of dance in building social knowledge, with particular attention paid to current methodological innovations and what has led up to these practices. It is important to bear in mind that this is a very new innovation and we are in the preliminary stages of watching it develop. Although dance-based methods cannot simply follow performance-based models, the wealth of methodological exploration of performance-based methods can be called on as dance-based methods emerge. In the following article Mary Beth Cancienne and Celeste Snowber, two of the most prominent scholars in the field of dance and movement studies, review some of the major theoretical and methodological innovations in movement studies and provide individual and collaborative examples of how this methodology can be employed.

DISCUSSION QUESTIONS AND ACTIVITIES

1. What is the relationship between theoretical advances in embodiment research and methodological innovation in dance and movement research?

2. How can social researchers employ dance as a methodological device? What strategies are available for using dance as a data collection method? How can dance and movement be used in multimethod research? How can dance be used as a representational form? What are the potential advantages and disadvantages of this approach?

3. For this activity, try working with LMA, aimed at systematically studying movement. Get a video recording of professional dance (any genre), develop a coding procedure based on LMA, as reviewed in this chapter, and code the data. What does this method draw your attention to? What have you learned from this process?

SUGGESTED READINGS

Bagley, C., & Cancienne, M. (Eds.). (2002). *Dancing the data.* New York: Peter Lang.

This edited volume covers many topics pertaining to arts and social research, including readings about dance and social research by renowned scholars.

Williams, D. (1991, 2004). *Anthropology and the dance: Ten lectures.* Urbana and Chicago: University of Illinois Press.

This book offers a wide range of anthropological explanations for why people dance.

SUGGESTED WEBSITES AND JOURNALS

Journal of Dance Education
   www.jmichaelryan.com/JODE/jode-ad.html

Articles cover the range of dance education in all settings, including early childhood and preschool, K–12, higher education, private studio, special education and disabled persons, and children at risk. Articles address teaching methods and practices; curriculum and sequential learning; the aesthetic and creative process; use of higher-order thinking skills and problem solving; standards at the national, state, and local levels; assessments; professional preparation and teacher training; and interdisciplinary education.

Research in Dance Education
   www.tandf.co.uk/journals/titles/14647893.asp

This journal publishes research in dance education that is relevant to an international audience of learners and teachers. Topics covered include all phases of education, preschool to higher education and beyond; teaching and learning in dance, theory, and practice; new methodology and technology; and professional dance artists in education. This journal also has special sections. The Perspectives section aims to republish significant research that may no longer be available in print, and the Dancelines section showcases outstanding student writing.

Electric Journal of Folklore
www.folklore.ee/folklore

The *Electronic Journal of Folklore* publishes original academic articles in folklore studies, comparative mythological research, cultural anthropology, and related fields. The journal is issued in print and in a full free online version (*www.folklore.ee/folklore*). The electronic journal includes video and audio samples.

Journal of Folklife
www.folklifestudies.org.uk

Founded in 1961, the Society of Folklife Studies is the only organization in Britain that brings together curators, historians, geographers, musicologists, linguists, and many other people to explore the regional identity of the British Isles and beyond. Areas of consideration include traditional crafts, costume and material culture, vernacular architecture, landscape studies, and custom and tradition.

Journal of Folklore Research
www.indiana.edu/~jofr/about.php

Founded in 1964, the *Journal of Folklore Research* is published by the Department of Folklore and Ethnomusicology at Indiana University. Until 1983 it was known as the *Journal of the Folklore Institute.* The journal is devoted to the study of the world's traditional creative and expressive forms and provides an international forum for current theory and research among scholars of folklore and related fields.

Qualitative Inquiry

This peer-reviewed journal publishes a range of articles dealing with innovative qualitative methods, including many arts-based practices. Many articles about dance and social research have appeared in this journal.

Anthropology and Dance Website of Interest
www.csap.bham.ac.uk/resources/project_reports/findings/ShowFinding.asp?id=57

Two anthropology graduates carried out a nationwide survey of lecturers and students in the anthropology of art to determine what they would like to see on a website dedicated to the anthropology of art. The results informed the creation of this site.

NOTES

1. Bernie Warren (1993) also suggests several reasons why dance is beneficial to the ill. On a philosophical level, the body serves as an instrument that is used to communicate thoughts, feelings, and a range of information (p. 58) (as explored in-depth by symbolic interactionists in the social and behavioral sciences). In this vein, children learn about the world by moving their bodies through it and interacting with their environment (p. 58). Therefore, experimenting with dance and movement is a way of learning about the self. Warren further asserts the sick and disabled need a means of self-expression to aide their well-being, broadly conceived. There are physical, bodily benefits as well. Warren suggests that dance and movement can help control the muscle spasms experienced by people with cerebral palsy and can also strengthen fine and gross motor skills, neurological functions, and circulatory regulation (p. 59).

2. Kingma posits that that the social gendering of dance often excludes boys from participating in this form of artistic expression—often viewed as a "feminine" activity. However, as Kingma points out, dance provides a medium for self-expression and can foster confidence. Kingma uses the example of one boy who was very shy until he discovered dance, through which he cultivated a positive self-concept. Now an adult, he is a youth pastor in Australia who uses dance to help young people nurture positive self-esteem.

REFERENCES

Bagley, C., & Cancienne, M. B. (2002). Educational research and intertextual forms of (re)presentation. In C. Bagley & M. B. Cancienne (Eds.), *Dancing the data* (pp. 3–32). New York: Peter Lang.

Beck, R. J., Martinez, M. E., & Lires, M. (1999). The application of an expert model of interpretive skill to a multicultural–multimedia system on ethnic dance. *Studies in Art Education, 40*(2), 162–179.

Blumenfeld-Jones, D. S. (2002). If I could have said it, I would have. In C. Bagley & M. B. Cancienne (Eds.), *Dancing the data* (pp. 90–104). New York: Peter Lang.

Bordo, S. (1989). Feminism, postmodernism, and gender skepticism. In L. Nicholson (Ed.), *Feminism/postmodernism* (pp. 133–156). New York: Routledge.

Burstin, F. (2004, September 4). New beat to speech skills. *Courier Mail* (Brisbane, Australia), p. L13.

Clark-Rapley, E. (1999). Dancing bodies: Moving beyond Marxian views of human activity, relations and consciousness. *Journal for the Theory of Social Behavior, 29*(2), 89–108.

Daly, A. (1988). Movement analysis: Piecing together the puzzle. *Drama Review, 32*(4), 40–52.

Foucault, M. (1976). Power as knowledge. In R. Hurley (Trans.), *The history of sexuality: Vol. 1. An introduction* (pp. 92–102). New York: Vintage Books.

Freedman, D. C. (1991). Gender signs: An effort/shape analysis of Romanian couple dances. *Studia Musicologica Academiae Scientiarum Hungaricae,* *33*(1), 335–345.

Grosz, E. (1994). *Volatile bodies: Toward a corporeal feminism.* Bloomington: Indiana University Press.

Henry, R. (2000). Introduction—anthropology of dance. *Australian Journal of Anthropology, 11*(3), 253–260.

Hesse-Biber, S. N., & Leavy, P. (2005). *The practice of qualitative research.* Thousand Oaks, CA: Sage.

Kim, Y. (2004, September 12). Exploring ancient multi-dimensional healing methods. *Sarasota Herald-Tribune,* p. BS4.

Kingma, J. (2004, April 7). Using dance to help boys find out who they are. *Canberra Times,* p. A25.

Merleau-Ponty, M. (1962). *Phenomenology of perception* (C. Smith, Trans.). London: Routledge & Kegan Paul.

Picard, C. (2000). Patterns of expanding consciousness in midlife women. *Nursing Science Quarterly, 13*(2), 150–157.

Picart, C. J. (2002). Dancing through different worlds: An autoethnography of the interactive body and virtual emotions in ballroom dance. *Qualitative Inquiry, 8*(3), 348–361.

Sklar, D. (2000). Reprise: On dance ethnography. *Dance Research Journal, 32*(1), 70–77.

Snowber, C. (2002). Bodydance: Enfleshing soulful inquiry through improvisation. In C. Bagley & M. B. Cancienne (Eds.), *Dancing the data* (pp. 20–33). New York: Peter Lang.

Spry, T. (2006). Performing autoethnography: An embodied methodological praxis. In S. N. Hesse-Biber & P. Leavy (Eds.), *Emergent methods in social research* (pp. 706–732). Thousand Oaks, CA: Sage.

Stinson, S. W. (1995). Body of knowledge. *Educational Theory, 45*(1), 43–54.

Stinson, S. W. (1998). Seeking a feminist pedagogy for children's dance. In S. Shapiro (Ed.), *Dance, power, and difference: Critical and feminist perspectives in dance education* (pp. 23–48). Champaign, IL: Human Kinetics.

Stinson, S. W. (2004). My body/myself: Lessons from dance education. In L. Bresler (Ed.), *Knowing bodies, moving minds: Toward embodied teaching and learning.* London: Kluwer Academic.

Warren, B. (Ed.). (1993). *Using the creative arts in therapy: A practical introduction.* New York: Routledge.

Yaman, E. (2003, September 6). Music as medicine reaches a crescendo. *The Weekend Australian,* p. B55.

Writing Rhythm
Movement as Method

Mary Beth Cancienne
Celeste N. Snowber

> We only believe those thoughts which have been conceived
> not in the brain but in the whole body.
>
> —W. B. Yeats

The Body as the Site of Knowledge

We are moving researchers. Choreographing, dancing, and writing are integral to our professional lives as arts-based researchers. We use movement methods within the educational research process to pose critical questions; to connect with the emotions of participants; to understand theoretical concepts, the self as place of discovery; and to represent research through performance for an audience (Bagley & Cancienne, 2001). Dance is not only an expression of our research but also a form of inquiry into the research process. The choreographer/performer has long known that the choreographic process is one of sorting, sifting, editing, forming, making, and remaking; it's essentially an act of discovery. Combining dance, a kinesthetic form, and writing, a cognitive form, can forge relationships between body and mind, cognitive and affective knowing, and the intellect with physical vigor. Fundamental to integrating dance as part of the research process is the premise that the body is a site of knowledge (Abram, 1996; Friedman & Moon, 1997; Griffin, 1995; Mairs, 1989; Sheets-Johnstone, 1992).

The body is, no doubt, informed and inscribed by many political, social, and cultural discourses, which have legitimized the body in its relationship to knowledge. It has been therefore helpful to understanding the body from a variety of perspectives, including performance studies, dance therapy, semiotics, communication theory, and feminist studies. For too long, the polarities rooted in Cartesian dualism posited two distinct and mutually exclusive regions of human experience: mind and body. The evolution of these binary distinctions continues to be challenged, and there is now a wealth of criticism (Butler, 1993; Cataldi, 1993; Griffin, 1995; Grosz, 1994; Irigaray, 1992; Kristeva, 1980; Leder, 1990; McFague, 1993) that contributes to this major epistemological challenge. The terminology that inscribes the body brings us to descriptions of the corporeal body, the phenomenological body, the inscribed body, the politicized body, the signified body, the sexualized body—all of which have contributed both to our conceptualization of the body and its relationship to knowledge and to our understanding of how we inhabit our bodies and perceive others' bodies.

The Lived Experience

How we conceptualize the body intellectually is different from how we experience through dance the living, breathing, pulsing body from the inside out. For our purposes as researchers who are both dancers and academics, we draw on theoretical accounts of the body that describe the body from lived experience. We therefore draw on phenomenological curriculum research as well as autobiographical and narrative inquiry as models for integrating dance within the research process. Curriculum research that has drawn on the field of phenomenology (Husserl, 1970; Merleau-Ponty, 1964) has sought not so much to explain the world but rather to describe closely the ways in which we immediately experience an intimacy with the living world, attending to its myriad textures, sounds, flavors, and gestures. Phenomenological curriculum research has described the lived experience of the body as central to learning, being, knowing, and teaching, and such curriculum theorists as Max van Manen (1990), Madeleine Grumet (1988), Ted Aoki (1993), David Jardine (1998), William Pinar (1994), and Maxine Greene (1995) have made great strides in integrating these aspects into their writing. Phenomenological reflection on embodiment suggests that as individuals, we are subjects separated from the world or from others but that we have access to knowledge of the body only by living it (Grosz, 1994, p. 86). We extend this description to dancing.

There is a cautionary tale in viewing the body as only a text to be read. Although postmodern scholars have viewed the immediate act of dancing as a discourse for the purpose of reading and then writing about it, we also want our audiences to sweat, blush, jubilate, and lament while watching a performance. As dancers, it is our limbs, torsos, gestures, pelvis, hips, legs, and hands that excavate the nexus of knowledge, insight, and understanding. Our dancing bodies become a place where we can cultivate a sense of embodiment in an age in which analysis and fragmentation often thwart us in recognizing and exploring the meaning of the ordinary, bodily acts of our lives. It is these ordinary acts of life that we research through our dance: the meaning of engaging in work, the human capacity for longing and desire, the integration of intellectual ideas and physicality, and the relationship between culture and identity. The approach of integrating the choreographic process as central to research begins to shift the perception that we have bodies to the reality that we are bodies. We hope that the knowledge intrinsic to the choreographic process can contribute to the larger paradigm of how research becomes a continued place of discovery, one that includes a physical apprehension and expression of the world.

Choreography and Performance

Choreography, the art of dance, and everyday movement provide a rhythmic pattern, a system of meaningful motions of the body that can communicate an interpretation of the world in which we live. Each person's movement schema expresses social and cultural meanings. Sklar (1994) argued that "movement embodies socially constructed cultural knowledge in which corporeality, emotion, and abstraction are intertwined" (p. 12). At the same time, Albright (1997) argued that bodies not only represent social constructions of gender, race, and sexuality but also embody a somatic identity (the experience of one's physicality). Albright concluded that coupling cultural identity and somatic identity enables the dancer both to reenact and challenge his or her identity. As arts-based researchers, we explore how we have been socially constructed through our bodies as well as how the physicality of our technique and lived experience moves us beyond our social constructions. This exploration is important to the development of an educational movement researcher. Other articles that explore choreography and dance in teaching and research include Blumenfeld-Jones (1995), Stinson (1995), Davenport and Forbes (1997), Snowber and Gerofsky (1998), Apol and Kambour (1999), Cancienne (1999), Bagley and Cancienne (2001), Cancienne and Megibow (2001), Markula and Denison (2001), and Spry (2001).

In the practices of researching and teaching, we pose the methods-based questions, How do we write performance? How do our performances write us? As a way of writing these performances and reflecting on how these performances can illuminate aspects of the research process, Cancienne explores the activities of domestic chores influenced by her Cajun culture by choreographing a piece titled "Women's Work." Snowber explains how she explored the relationship between math and dance in "Beyond the Span of My Limbs: Gesture, Number, and Infinity."

Implicit in these performances is the qualitative aspect of "self as instrument" (Eisner, 1998). Instead of considering the body as only an instrument or tool, as it often is, we would like to encourage a broader view of the body as a locus of discovery (Halprin, 1995, 2000). Therefore, we use the phrase *self as a place of discovery* in our discussion. After describing the performances, we reflect on them by focusing on the questions they have posed for us. Finally, we discuss how these interpretations influence how we "see" arts-based research.

Cancienne's Voice

Women's Work

Descriptive writing on dance and performance is limited. Mostly, there are critiques of choreographers' works with brief excerpts of performances. Goldberg (1997) suggested that choreographers not leave the job only to critics. Instead, she suggested, the choreographer can and should do some of the work. Therefore, I begin by describing a piece I choreographed titled "Women's Work." I then reflect on how I have reenacted social constructions of gender and also moved beyond these constructions. Describing my own choreography, embracing it, and finally challenging it are important steps in the development of the self as a place of discovery within the research process. Gottschild (1997) was in agreement with my own personal claims. She wrote, "I find that choreography and the dancing body play a role in shaping my approach to research" (p. 167). In this sense, both the researcher and the choreographer use kinesthetic and cognitive approaches to formulate ideas and move beyond stereotypes.

According to Highwater (1992), ritual is primary in making meaning within a culture and "produced by all peoples still in touch with the capacity to express themselves in metaphor" (p. 14). "Women's Work" explores ritual through my own cultural heritage (Cajun), in that I transform my past experience of doing daily domestic chores as a child into a metaphoric idiom. The music chosen for this dance is also metaphorical. The Baka Forest People of Southeast Cameroon play water drums for "Women's Work." I chose this music because it has associations to women's physical experience while using water to wash, scrub, and clean; drums, symbolic of the heartbeat, represent women's varying levels of breath while working.

The 4-minute CD, titled *Water Drums I* (Heart of the Forest, 1993), begins. The three dancers, ranging in age from 32 to 50, are barefoot and wear black pants with multicolored loose shirts that hang below their waists. Their long-sleeved shirts are extremely loose to accentuate the flow and suspension of the circular motions. As the water drums sound, the women enter one at a time. The first woman steps forward, taking proud, grandiose strides. She travels in a semicircle while succinctly sweeping one hand at a time up from the center of her torso to the side of her body. After six traveling sweeps, she turns, bends at the hips, sweeps the right hand past her right ankle as the left leg swings back and upward, and then sweeps her right arm upward to an extended arm as her left leg sweeps down. Next, she arrogantly sweeps her right hand to the left across the front of her face and over her shoulder as she sharply turns her head to the right in the opposite direction. At this moment, the second woman enters.

After all three women enter the dance space, the "work" phase begins. This section is at times monotonous and repetitive, almost trancelike, but is mixed with energetic bursts and athletic jumps, as a way of challenging the audience not to fall too deeply and thus to fight against the trance. The dancers use hands, feet, torsos, figure eights, semicircles, and forward and backward circles to depict stirring the pot, sweeping the floor, washing the dishes, and making the bed. Each dancer performs these movements in a prescribed sequence and at a different level. For instance, when one dancer is washing in figure eights on a medium plane, the second dancer is sweeping by swinging her leg and arm at a low level (horizontally on the floor), while the third dancer is stirring the batter at a higher point by swinging her arm back and forth like a windmill.

In the third section of the performance, the women turn and face each other inside the circle, pause, look at each other, and then begin to wash clothes. The circle of washing then moves to a circle of internal struggles, depicted physically by having the women contract their pelvises with their arms strapped to their sides while on their knees, lowering their upper bodies back toward the floor while their heads lean over their right shoulders. These movements are variations on Graham contractions performed at different levels. The three women relate to each other through their movements, which is depicted by their dancing "in the round."

In the fourth section, the women return to doing their chores, and their movements are now expanded in height and width. At the end of each circular rotation of washing, cooking, and sweeping at a low, medium, and high level, the dancers elongate their movements to full-fledged jumps, turns, and leaps. The semicircles, circles, and figure eights of their chores are now leaps as well as jumps in wide first and second positions with arms extended overhead and to the side.

In the finale, the women repeat the same movements as in the opening section, except that this time the dancers stand in a straight line facing first the center of the audience, then the right side of the audience, and finally the left side of the audience. With these final movements, dancers announce that they are done with their chores for the day. Finally, the heavily breathing dancers slowly melt down to the floor while giving their weight to each other for support. The lights narrow on the three women as Kathy Glover, poet and middle school language arts teacher, reads a poem titled "All Life Is Richness of Rhythm."

The substance for "Women's Work" consists of the daily chores (e.g., stirring the pot, washing the clothes, and sweeping the floor) that I participated in as a child in my home. Of course, these dance movements are metaphorical, as there were no props used onstage. As such, the substance highlights the theme of gender. The movements are associated with domestic activities that have traditionally been performed by women. This piece also focuses on the relationships that develop between women who work together. By moving separately and "in the round," the dancers enact a sense of independence and community.

"Women's Work" was one of three performance works for a show titled *Dance Talk Two,* which was presented for two weekends at McGuffey Arts Center in Charlottesville, Virginia, in 1999. The audience members were mostly artists, dancers, university students, and community members. The overall theme of the show focused on connections among movement, language, and spaces where movement stands alone. After the 1-hour show, the performers/choreographers engaged in a postperformance dialogue. During this dialogue, one audience member, a dancer, stated that the music was energetic, the movements big, and the dance culturally ethnic and primitive. She added, "It was an ancient feeling. The image was of women down by the river pounding the clothes against the rocks." A mechanical engineering student said that he felt both emotional and physical responses during the finale. He wanted to know how a physical performance evokes these charged feelings. One explanation is that our bodies are contours of our emotions. Borrowing from Brazilian folklore theory, Young (1994) stated that emotions have "substance, weight, and volume. ... Emotion issues from the body and enters into other bodies; it has direction or can be directed and it affects bodily tissues" (p. 7). What we experience when watching a dance performance affects the intricate balance of our bodies and those around us. Highwater (1992) explained, "Because of the inherent contagion of motion, the dancer is able to convey nonverbally, even nonsymbolically, the most intangible experiences, ideas, and feelings" (p. 24). The emotions revealed in the "Women's Work" dancers' sharp movements make audience members alert and stand in contrast to the sense of monotony and tranquility of repetition in the "work phrase" and "washing phrase." Quick changes between low and high stance and sharp angular motion add to the rush of emotion. This contrast wakens the audience from the trance of circles and plunges them into the world of suspense and attention.

"Women's Work" is based on the traditional modern dance technique of Graham (release and contraction) and Horton. I initially studied these techniques in the late 1980s while on scholarship at the Alvin Ailey American Dance Theater in New York City. Ailey's style and approach to dance are very different from those at most schools of dance. For Ailey, although technique is important, the dancer's face and body must be expressive and unique; his company is not interested in producing cookie-cutter dancers. In addition, the traditional stereotype of the tall, thin dancer is not the Ailey norm; instead, different body shapes, sizes, and heights are a central part of his repertoire. Furthermore, because my goal is to explore the lived experience of many different types of women, my interpretation must be multidimensional to represent the diversity of female experience.

"Women's Work" is radically different from the other pieces that I have choreographed in the past. Usually, I choreographed literary pieces, curriculum theory writings, or autobiographical reflections. "Women's Work" is not an interpretation of a written text; rather, its inspiration comes from the body and its inherent connection to water and drums. While choreographing "Women's Work," I read Dewey's (1934) *Art as Experience,* which inspired me to focus on both meaning and form in art making.

After reflecting on "Women's Work" and reading texts from cultural studies in dance (Albright, 1997; Desmond, 1997) as well as books on my own culture (Ancelet, Edwards, & Pitre, 1991), I now understand how "Women's Work" speaks to me in ways that reading and writing alone do not. Because the researcher interprets and uses the self as a place of discovery for judging what is important in the data (Eisner, 1998), the best place to begin my own research is to dance. As a way of listening to my inner voice, dance is a corporeal way of knowing, a different way of seeing, questioning, and challenging. For researchers who have danced for most of their lives, the body becomes an articulate surface for exploration. What I have discovered through "Women's Work" is that people from oral cultures or diverse language cultures can cross over to academic culture without leaving their oral cultures behind. My process of using choreography and self-reflexive writing is an approach of transitioning without giving up one for the other.

Burton (2001) defined culture as everything that can be learned. Often, what I learned as a child growing up in my ethnic culture differs greatly from the learning that has taken place as an adult breaking into the culture of academia. Highwater (1992) wrote,

> At the core of everyone's culture is a package of beliefs which every child learns and which has been culturally determined long in advance of his or her birth. The world is rendered coherent by our description of it. What we see when we speak of reality is simply that preconception. (p. 33)

Choreography represents a flexible, meaningful way of exploring these preconceptions to integrate my past with my present. It acts as a mirror to my culturally inscribed body. Because the body is socially constructed, it communicates social practices and cultural meanings through voice, gesture, and movement (Desmond, 1997). In essence, the body is not simply flesh and bones; instead, it is a living enactment of culture and social beliefs. Albright (1997) wrote, "Because dance comprises the daily technical training of the dancer's body as well as the final choreographic production, dance can help us trace the complex negotiations between somatic experience and the cultural representation   between the body and identity" (p. xiv). Embedded in my choreography are social practices from childhood as well as articulated movements from practiced dance techniques. For instance, an important value in the Cajun culture is the sharing of the workload among the young and old. Children learn early on to become responsible for chores (Ancelet et al., 1991), which was certainly true within my own upbringing. The act of making my bed before going to school in the morning was a domestic practice that I incorporated into "Women's Work." In a sense, these practices become identities that I bring to my research.

In "Women's Work," I romanticize, play with, and question idealized images of the domesticated woman. For instance, we see the idealization of chores in "Women's Work" when one woman is washing using figure eight motions, swinging her hips and arms. The dancer looks as if she is doing a towel dance at the *fais do-do* (street dance) on Saturday night rather than doing hard physical labor.

At first glance, romanticizing chores in "Women's Work" does not move beyond the stereotype that women should be domestic homemakers. In this sense, "Women's Work" is limiting and does not recognize the diverse roles women play on the bayou. On the other hand, the physicality of the dance itself moves beyond the stereotype that women and in particular Cajun women are shy, weak, helpless, and fragile. This piece also challenges the stereotype that only young women should dance in performance. The women dancing are not young dancers. Instead, they are aged, healthy, and strong. Finally, this piece explores the dignity that is embedded in the ritual of domestic work. Because "Women's Work" is in progress, I am still experimenting with gender roles, especially as they transcend daily chores. This interrogation of my work is one example of how choreography influences my research process. Within the research process, it is important to see participants, or dancers, as multidimensional and diverse.

Traditionally, academics, not the participants themselves, have studied oral cultures. In today's research community, the participant is becoming ever more the researcher. I am not alone in my experiential approach to choreography; indeed, many researchers connect strongly to their traditional or family cultures, which are rich in song, dance, music, and storytelling. Researchers should continue developing arts-based methods that enable new, vibrant, and diverse models for its heterogeneous research community. Choreography and self-reflexive writing (as shown in this article) allow me to move beyond the constraints of academic writing: By recognizing the culture of my childhood, I can more effectively communicate my research findings while illustrating my ideas and findings to a scholarly audience. "Women's Work" is one tapestry of childhood influences that I bring to the writing table as an arts-based researcher whose place of discovery is centered in the self.

Snowber's Voice

Beyond the Span of My Limbs: Gesture, Number, and Infinity

"Beyond the Span of My Limbs: Gesture, Number, and Infinity" was a performance piece that I researched and performed with a colleague, Susan Gerofsky, who is a mathematics educator. We came together, dancer and mathematician, to inquire into the relationships between math and dance and, more specifically, to find the connections between the experience of the finite and infinite in math, dance, and art. The domains of both mathematics and dance share a fascination with the establishment and the breaking of boundaries in space and time, and with the exploration of the quest for transcendence. The dancer captures glimpses of the inexpressible, unknowable elements of lived experience and gives voice to the concerns of both mathematicians and dancers. This 45-minute performance piece incorporates modern dance, creative movement, improvisation, music, poetry, readings from our own writings and those of others, and audience participation.

In performance, "Beyond the Span of My Limbs" becomes an embodied space within which we inquire into the lived relationships of space and time, and the visceral connections between longing, desire, and limits (Irigaray, 1992; Vilenkin, 1995). This piece was performed in a variety of venues, including three educational conferences, a faculty of education, movement education classes, and a high school. High school students had a chance to view the performance and reflect/write on the process, a process that allowed them to examine their own questions of the relationships between performance art, dance, and the philosophical questions of limits/space/boundaries in their own lives.

Mathematics is often seen as disembodied and conceptual, an abstraction of an abstraction (Moritz, 1942; Rotman, 1993). Our schooling has traditionally compartmentalized the mental and conceptual apart from the physical and the expressive, keeping mathematics, art, and movement strictly separated (Snowber & Gerofsky, 1998). Yet our mathematical intuitions and imaginations start from simple concepts of counting, an activity that is tied to physical objects and physical understandings. In our dance, we literally use counting to engender movement, counting on each other's toes, fingers, and knuckles and performing children's games of counting. It can be difficult to fully comprehend the abstract other than through our bodies. We reach toward the infinite with the living and finite—with limbs, torsos, hips, fingertips, and the rhythm of our breath (Snowber & Gerofsky, 1998).

As I personally danced the concepts of math, I was surprised to find how much relationship there was to math and my own background in choreography. As math has forms, rules, and pattern, so does choreography in its use of composition, design, pattern, repetition, shape, space, and quality of movement. I have felt in the past that the discipline of math had little relationship to my life experiences, but in dancing "Beyond the Span of My Limbs," I became aware of how deeply embedded it is in the workings of my embodied self. I could make geometric shapes with my body and physically "understand" those shapes. As a result, I continue to incorporate angles, curves, spirals, and circles into my aesthetic designs. Moreover, the finiteness of my body is the very matter that reaches,

pushes, extends, pulls, stretches, contracts, and glides into the infinite-
ness of space.

Central to "Beyond the Span of My Limbs" is exploring the notion
of limits with the body. Before choreographing this dance, I had written
about the notion of longing and desire in my doctoral dissertation, which
was focused on a poetics of embodiment and its relationship to knowing,
being, living, and teaching (Snowber, 1998). During the period of doctoral studies I injured my knee, and a sports medicine specialist informed
me that I may never dance again. I had recently made a commitment to
myself that I would dance as long as my body was able. After all, Martha
Graham (1991), the pioneer modern dancer, danced till age 90! Dance is
primary to my well-being and a continual source of invitation to enter
life fully. The thought of not dancing would represent a profound sense
of death to both body and soul.

I decided that I would still dance through this injury, using a chair
as a tangible object that would serve both as a limit and a support. The
chair allowed me to bear weight, almost as another leg, allowing me to
lean on it, fall over it, rock in it, extend a leg into the air, contract and
release from its wooden form, and even throw it. For a year, I improvised
dancing on various chairs (against my doctor's advice) and simultaneously wrote chapters for my dissertation on the nature of longing and
desire. What culminated from my improvising dance on chairs was a solo
on the chair, which was incorporated into the piece "Beyond the Span of
My Limbs" and danced in a variety of other performance venues.

By incorporating the chair into my notion of myself as a dancer, I
explored the relationship of limits, in which longing became visible in
artistic form. My body used gravity and levity as I pressed against the
wooden frame of the chair, arched into space from its weight, collapsed in
its security, and even kicked it abruptly across the floor. At another point,
I caressed the chair, rocked in its secure hold, and stood on it with my
upper back and arms arched backward, extending my spine to the limits
of upward space. Bulgarian chants sounded in the background, echoing
the laments and longing of a torso leaning inward and outward at the
same time.

As I performed this piece over and over again, I was invited to understand limits and infinity in ways that no other discipline could teach me.
It is within mathematical inquiry that the concepts of limit and the infinite are interconnected. The geometric boundary of the chair became a
point to access beyond the finite, and for a moment, dancer and audience
could touch transcendence. The solo on the chair was only one 4-min-
ute dance within the larger 45-minute performance piece of "Beyond the
Span of My Limbs," but I use this particular dance as the point of refer-

ence for the place where my research questions were most challenged, explored, and opened up.

Performing the dance solo with the chair deepened my understanding of the relationship between math and dance, but even more, it reframed my conceptions of the notions of limits. I have not always thought of limits as places of possibilities but places of obstacle, something to be jumped, danced, or skipped over. I certainly could not have seen how a place of extension and openness could be sustained and fostered by a limit. The constraint of having a knee injury motivated me to use the chair as a support. What emerged from this experience was an entirely new movement language, which I perhaps never would have found otherwise. As an artist or dancer, I find it easy to rely on the predictable, the language that is familiar. By encountering the limit of a chair, I was forced to create movements in a way I never would have imagined, as I had to adjust my body to not leaping, jumping, hopping, or landing hard on my feet. As I had intellectually explored the notion of longing as it related to desire, my whole body had the opportunity to wrestle, stay with, and eventually delight in the limit. The limit transformed me to a place of support for my body and shifted my own perception of limits in life experience. Through the boundary, I am invited into a whole new language of dance—one that fits my midlife body, which has physical limitations and yet more choreographic possibilities.

The question that I had explored within my doctoral research was how can we bring desire, passion, and longing to the root of the acts of living and being? Although I was steeped in the literature of poststructural feminists such as Luce Irigaray (1992), who spoke of the limit becoming the wound or the place for the sky to open up, it was only in repeatedly performing a dance from the chair that I began to touch the relationship between pain and release, transcendence and immanence, finiteness and infinity. The beginning of bringing desire to living and being is to notice and attend to the places of struggle and pain. My dancing, in turn, affected my writing both in its form and the emergent theme of paradox as central to embodiment. This dance continues to be a teacher to me as I look at every situation with new eyes, reserving judgment and allowing for the limit to be a place of new birth in my work as a dancer, educator, and researcher.

This dance speaks to the audience in their responses of how it allows them to connect to their own longings and desires, even the desire to articulate lament. During this piece, I am sitting on the chair, my pelvis contracted and my upper body swinging over in circular movements, flexing feet, and dancing a litany for what is lost. I dance absence and presence, loss and anger, longing and mourning, and eventually, my limbs move daringly into release and strength. Audiences often find the articulation of these stages of longing to be a place for them to attend to the places of pain or desertion in their own lives. The performer kinesthetically gives audience members the opportunity to honor their own experiences and acknowledge its place in their own educational journeys.

Cancienne's and Snowber's Voices

Interplay

As we speak of the interplay between writing and dance, it is important to remember that writing begins not only when we put pen to paper or fingers to the keyboard, but also in the way we are consciously embodied—the way we breathe, think, and feel in our bodies. Writing is essentially attention. Part of the researcher's responsibility within the inquiry process is to pay "attention to particulars" (Eisner, 1998, p. 38). Therefore, as researchers, we must notice the details of our lives and access the nooks and crannies of our experiences and perceptions. Attentiveness is not something we do only with the mind but can be an act of "bodily attending," a way to be present to the physicality of the textures around us: sound, gesture, smell, sight—the vowels of the physical world (Snowber, 1997). Therefore, writing becomes not just a recording of details but a process by which we are awakened to the details of experience. In the same way, dancing becomes not just a recording of knowledge but a process by which we are awakened to new insights.

Even though we use writing as a method of reflection, one question that we ask is, How can we access a way of writing from the body, a way in which theory meets practice so that the deep listening to life actually spills over from blood to ink? Hélène Cixous (1993) said, "Writing is not arriving; most of the time it's not arriving. One must go on foot with the body" (p. 65). Dance allows us to taste the grammar of the gut, the alphabet of the bones, the etymology of the pelvis. The process of dancing, choreographing, improvising, and reworking movement ultimately opens up a place to drop into the belly, allowing poetic and artistic knowing to sing, dance, and write out of our bodies. Writing from the body becomes an interaction between knowing and being, ontology and epistemology, and the ordinary and the extraordinary.

The orality of spoken language is centered on breath, which shapes the rhythm, intonation, speed, and resonance of sound. Breath can bring us closer to the body's textures and rhythms, as has been convincingly articulated by David Abram (1996): "As we reacquaint ourselves with our breathing bodies, then the perceived world itself begins to shift and transform" (p. 63). The body begins to let go of tension when we attend to breath. This release opens up the capacity to perceive the world with freshness. The practice of returning to breath as a way of attentiveness and remembering has been stated by dance educators (Blom & Chaplin, 1988; Cheney, 1989; Hanna, 1988). In the fertile place of breathing fully, one is invited to hear the words and vibrations in the body and can call the mind to attend more deeply to the questions of the body.

As movement inquirers within arts-based approaches to qualitative research, we write to articulate the meanings of our movements and methods. Moreover, we write to illustrate how this approach adds to the existing body of educational research. Currently, journal representations privilege the printed word over other forms of expression. Movement methods, although represented through journal articles, should use other forms such as multimedia as legitimate representations of arts-based research methods. Once this technology is accepted in professional circles, an array of intertextual forms can be used to relay valuable information. In the book *Dancing the Data* (Bagley & Cancienne, 2002), and the companion CD-ROM *Dancing the Data, Too* (Cancienne & Bagley, 2002), the artistic researchers represent their educational research through dance, theater, poetry, music, collage, and photography. Although both written text and multimedia text are representational forms, these media provide a place for arts-based inquiry to be expressed more fully.

Publishing in journals and multimedia to represent movement methods such as choreography can enhance qualitative inquiry by connecting with people's natural understanding of breath, voice, rhythm, and emotion. These are all inherent parts of any human experience but are commonly overlooked and thus taken for granted outside the purview of cognitive experience. An understanding of everyday movements can contribute to a more holistic awareness of the lives of students, teachers, school administrators, and ourselves, the researchers who observe, interview, interpret, and represent these explorations.

Finally, there are dangers to movement-based research that must be noted. Bodies have weight, scents, voices, personalities, emotions, rhythms, and energies that inevitably collide and resist. Bodies in education have been silenced, abused, overpowered, and used in ways that are unsafe and destructive (Brunner, 1996; Grumet, 1988). We also must be sensitive to the ways that the behavioral scientists and work environments have used bodies historically. We must not use movement methods as a way to further restrict bodies in our school system. We are more interested in using the body to release the tension, understand relationships of self and other, and ultimately to heal bodies that are silenced, stressed, and restricted in ways that are unhealthy.

Take, for example, a space in every school, its hallways. Many educators have yet to understand and value the hallways as places of interaction that can provide insights into students' lives. Perhaps through the application of movement methods in qualitative research, we will be able to interpret the students' body language exhibited in the relationships they form, the questions they ask, their rhythms in walking, their hand gestures, and their facial expressions. As arts-based researchers, we strive to understand what the students' improvisational hallway movement stories, or speaking dances, are saying and how adults can make meaning of their choreography, to glean information that will enhance student–teacher and student–student relationships (McLauren, 1999).

Artists, dancers, and performers know what it means to integrate the body as a place of unfolding learning. Maxine Sheets-Johnstone (1999), dance scholar, asserted that "thinking in movement is foundational to being a body" (p. 494). Understanding our bodies and movement is, therefore, an essential part of our existence (Markula & Denison, 2001, p. 427). Our intent, then, in integrating dance/movement within qualitative inquiry is to provide a place for researchers to teach, perceive, and transform education in ways that are overlooked—for it is in the process of movement method research that bodily-based theoretical frameworks can enlarge educational research.

References

Abram, D. (1996). *The spell of the sensuous: Perception and language in a more-than-human world*. New York: Pantheon.

Albright, A. C. (1997). *Choreographing difference: The body and identity in contemporary dance*. Middletown, CT: Wesleyan University Press.

Ancelet, B. J., Edwards, J., & Pitre, G. (1991). *Cajun country*. Jackson: University of Mississippi Press.

Aoki, T. (1993). Legitimizing lived curriculum: Toward a curricular landscape of multiplicity. *Journal of Curriculum and Supervision, 8*(3), 255–258.

Apol, L., & Kambour, T. (1999). Telling stories through writing and dance: An intergenerational project. *Language Arts, 77*(2), 106–117.

Bagley, C., & Cancienne, M. B. (2001). Educational research and intertextual forms of (re)presentation: The case for dancing the data. *Qualitative Inquiry, 7*(2), 221–237.

Bagley, C., & Cancienne, M. B. (Eds.). (2002). *Dancing the data*. New York: Peter Lang.

Blom, L. A., & Chaplin, L. T. (1988). *The moment of movement: Dance improvisation*. Pittsburgh, PA: University of Pittsburgh Press.

Blumenfeld-Jones, D. S. (1995). Dance as a mode of research representation. *Qualitative Inquiry, 4*, 391–401.

Brunner, D. D. (1996). Silent bodies: Miming those killing norms of gender. *Journal of Curriculum Studies, 12*(1), 9–15.

Burton, J. (2001). *Culture and the human body: An anthropological perspective.* Prospect Heights, IL: Waveland.

Butler, J. (1993). *Bodies that matter: On the discursive limits of "sex."* New York: Routledge.

Cancienne, M. B. (1999). The gender gaze: Rethinking gender through performance. *Journal of Curriculum Theorizing, 15*(2), 167–175.

Cancienne, M. B., & Bagley, C. (Eds.). (2002). *Dancing the data, too* [CD-ROM]. Charlottesville, VA: 2flydesigns.

Cancienne, M. B., & Megibow, A. (2001). The story of Anne: Movement as an educative text. *Journal of Curriculum Theory, 17*(2), 61–72.

Cataldi, S. L. (1993). *Emotion, depth, and flesh: A study of sensitive space.* Albany: State University of New York Press.

Cheney, G. (1989). *Basic concepts in modern dance: A creative approach.* Princeton, NJ: Dance Horizons.

Cixous, H. (1993). *Three steps on the ladder of writing.* New York: Routledge.

Davenport, D. R., & Forbes, C. A. (1997). Writing movement/dancing words: A collaborative pedagogy. *Education, 118*(2), 293–303.

Desmond, J. C. (1997). Embodying difference: Issues in dance and cultural studies. In J. C. Desmond (Ed.), *Meaning in motion. New cultural studies of dance* (pp. 29–54). Durham, NC: Duke University Press.

Dewey, J. (1934). *Art as experience.* New York: Perigee.

Eisner, E. (1998). *The enlightened eye: Qualitative inquiry and the enhancement of educational practice.* Upper Saddle River, NJ: Prentice Hall.

Friedman, L., & Moon, S. (Eds.). (1997). *Being bodies: Buddhist women on the paradox of embodiment.* Boston: Shambhala.

Goldberg, M. (1997). Homogenized ballerinas. In J. C. Desmond (Ed.), *Meaning in motion: New cultural studies of dance* (pp. 305–319). Durham, NC: Duke University Press.

Gottschild, B. D. (1997). Some thoughts on choreographing history. In J. C. Desmond (Ed.), *Meaning in motion: New cultural studies of dance* (pp. 167–177). Durham, NC: Duke University Press.

Graham, M. (1991). *Martha Graham: Blood memory.* New York: Washington Square Press.

Greene, M. (1995). *Releasing the imagination: Essays on education, the arts, and social change.* San Francisco: Jossey-Bass.

Griffin, S. (1995). *The eros of everyday life: Essays on ecology, gender and society.* New York: Anchor-Doubleday.

Grosz, E. (1994). *Volatile bodies: Toward a corporeal feminism.* Bloomington: Indiana University Press.

Grumet, M. (1988). *Bittermilk: Women and teaching.* Amherst: University of Massachusetts Press.

Halprin, A. (1995). *Moving toward life: Five decades of transformational dance.* Middletown, CT: Wesleyan University Press.

Halprin, A. (2000). *Dance as a healing art: Returning to health with movement and imagery.* Mendocino, CA: LifeRhythm.

Hanna, T. (1988). *Somatics: Reawakening the mind's control of movement, flexibility, and health.* Reading, MA: Addison-Wesley.

Heart of the Forest. (1993). *Water drums I* [CD]. Salem, MA: Rykodisc.

Highwater, J. (1992). *Dance: Rituals of experience* (3rd ed.). New York: Oxford University Press.

Husserl, E. (1970). *Cartesian meditations* (D. Cairns, Trans.). The Hague, The Netherlands: Nujhoff.

Irigaray, L. (1992). *Elemental passions* (J. Collie & J. Still, Trans.). London: Altone.

Jardine, D. (1998). *To dwell with a boundless heart: Essays in curriculum theory, hermeneutics and the ecological imagination.* New York: Lang.

Kristeva, J. (1980). *Desire in language: A semiotic approach to literature and art* (T. Gora, A. Jardine, & L. Roudiez, Trans.). New York: Columbia University Press.

Leder, D. (1990). *The absent body.* Chicago: University of Chicago Press.

Mairs, N. (1989). *Remembering the bone house: An erotics of place and space.* New York: Harper & Row.

Markula, P., & Denison, J. (2001). See Spot run: Movement as an object of textual analysis. *Qualitative Inquiry, 6*(3), 406–431.

McFague, S. (1993). *The body of God: An ecological theology.* Minneapolis, MN: Fortress Press.

McLauren, P. (1999). *Schooling as a ritual performance* (3rd ed.). New York: Rowman & Littlefield.

Merleau-Ponty, M. (1964). *The primacy of perception.* Evanston, IL: Northwestern University Press.

Moritz, R. E. (1942). *On mathematics and mathematicians (memorablia mathematica).* New York: Dover.

Pinar, W. F. (1994). *Autobiography, politics, and sexuality: Essays in curriculum theory, 1972–1992.* New York: Peter Lang.

Rotman, B. (1993). *Ad infinitum.* Stanford, CA: Stanford University Press.

Sheets-Johnstone, M. (Ed.). (1992). *Giving the body its due.* Albany: State University of New York Press.

Sheets-Johnstone, M. (1999). *The primacy of movement.* Philadelphia: Benjamin.

Sklar, D. (1994). Can bodylore be brought to its senses? *Journal of American Folklore, 107*(423), 9–22.

Snowber, C. (1997). Writing and the body. *Educational Insights, 4*(1). Available from *www.csci.educ.ubc.ca/publicaion/insights*

Snowber, C. (1998). *A poetics of embodiment: Cultivating an erotics of the every day.* Unpublished doctoral dissertation, Simon Fraser University, Burnaby, BC.

Snowber, C., & Gerofsky, S. (1998). Beyond the span of my limbs: Gesture, number and infinity. *Journal of Curriculum Theorizing, 15*(2), 39–48.

Spry, T. (2001). Performing autoethnography: An embodied methodological praxis. *Qualitative Inquiry, 7*(6), 706–732.

Stinson, S. (1995). Body of knowledge. *Educational Theory, 45*(1), 43–54.

van Manen, M. (1990). *Researching lived experience: Human science for an action-sensitive pedagogy.* London: Althouse.

Vilenkin, N. (1995). *In search of infinity* (A. Shenitzer, Trans.). Boston: Birkhauser.

Young, K. (1994). Whose body?: An introduction to bodylore. *Journal of American Folklore, 107*, 3–8.

CHAPTER 7

The Visual Arts

A picture can become for us a highway between a particular
thing and a universal feeling.
　　　　　　　　　—LAWREN HARRIS (in Fitzhenry, 1993, p. 45)

The power of the image, and its role in society, cannot be underesti-
mated. According to a popular expression, a picture is worth a thousand
words. This saying opens up two of the most paramount issues social
researchers consider as they use the visual arts in their knowledge-
building practices.

First, visual imagery does not represent a window onto the world,
but rather a created perspective. In photography, for example, photographs are popularly thought to "capture" and record some aspect of
the social world, neglecting the vantage point of the photographer, the
lens through which he or she looks, and the context in which the photograph is viewed. In this sense, visual art production can be likened to
journaling, a fact not lost on artists. In this regard, Cubist painter Pablo
Picasso noted that "painting is just another way of keeping a diary." Second, although visual imagery is created and the point of production is
inextricably bound to the art, visual art inherently opens up multiple
meanings that are determined not only by the artist but also the viewer
and the context of viewing (both the immediate circumstance and the
larger sociohistorical context).

Visual images are unique and can evoke particular kinds of emotional and visceral responses from their perceivers; they are typically
filed in the subconscious without the same conscious interpretive process

215

people engage in when confronted with a written text. Moreover, visual images occupy an elevated place in memory. This is evident when thinking about the collective memory of events, for example, how selected images come to represent the event, and how readily these images are available for mental recall. For example, when September 11th is mentioned Americans typically recall an image of New York's World Trade Center under some state of attack or destruction. In this regard, visual images are consumed differently than text and sound are. In short, visual images can be very powerful and lasting. The power of visual images is what has made them vitally important in our history and the ongoing trajectory of social progress, evident when we examine how images have been used to serve hegemonic authority and ideology as well as counterculture or otherwise resistive efforts.

As noted throughout this book, all art regardless of medium is a product of the time and place in which it is created, as well as the individual artist who is an embodied actor situated within the social order. The social context (cultural and institutional) in which visual art is produced historically constituted much of the draw for social scholars. In 1957 Mills encouraged anthropologists to use visual art in their research, positing it as a significant source of information within which researchers can discern patterns pertaining to individuals and society. He wrote that art acts as a barometer for change in society and labeled art "public objects" through which symbolic meaning is conveyed and "unconscious associations" created. Similarly, Warren (1993) labeled art a "record-keeper" and communicative device.

Visual art may serve as a vehicle for transmitting ideology while it can as effectively be used to challenge, dislodge, and transform outdated beliefs and stereotypes. In terms of the latter, visual images can be used as a powerful form of social and political resistance because the arts, and perhaps the visual arts in particular, always retain oppositional capabilities. Cultural norms and values, which change over time as they are contested and negotiated, shape the production of visual art. Furthermore, art is created in an economic context with market forces influencing changing definitions of "art," as well as their perceived value. Moreover, visual art is produced in an institutional context with various restraints, norms, pressures, and so forth influencing its production and circulation, as well as the value system within which it is judged.

The visual arts have long captivated both the public and scholars. As our society has become an increasingly visual one, with images appearing in multimedia in diverse settings from the mundane (consider modern advertising) to the "special" (museums created for the display of what is officially legitimized art), researchers have created various methods for incorporating the visual arts into their research, primarily as a source of data, analytical or interpretive tool, or representational form. In recent years social scientists have created a multitude of different visual arts-based methods, some of which are reviewed in this chapter.

In order to understand contemporary uses of visual art in research methodologies, it is necessary to consider the historical emergence of photography and documentary filmmaking in anthropology.

Visual Anthropology

Anthropologists have a history of using still and moving images as a source of data and representational vehicle. Hockings (2003) claims that films are a primary methodological tool in anthropology. Holm (2008) suggests that ethnographic films are the root of visual research methods. Although the continued (and expanded) use of moving images is important, given space constraints in this chapter I primarily focus on still images.

Collier and Collier (1986/1996) have been at the forefront of visual anthropology, delineating numerous strategies for using photography as a research method. Within these practices the camera serves as a research tool. Cameras allow researchers to gather data that is both selective and specific (1986/1996, pp. 9–10). Anthropologists often couple interviewing with photography from which they develop "photo essays," one approach to anthropological description (pp. 106–108). This approach can be applied to various ethnographic practices across the social sciences.

Influenced by this pioneering work, Holm (2008) notes three genres of visual images: (1) subject-produced images, (2) researcher-produced images, and (3) preexisting images. When researchers produce images it is vital to provide context, and Holm suggests using artist's statements as a model for how to accomplish this. Later in this chapter artist Maryjean Viano Crowe's visual art is accompanied by an artist statement as an example. Preexisting images may be used as "historical documents"; however, researchers need to be cautious as contextual information may be scarce.

As researchers consider the analysis of photographic data Collier and Collier warn that the goal should not be to "decode" or "translate" visual data into verbal data per se, but rather to build a bridge between the visual and the verbal (1986/1996, p. 169).

Drawing on earlier work by Collier and Collier, Malcolm Collier (2001) suggests a basic analysis model grounded in historical practices in visual anthropology. The analysis process involves four phases. First, observe the data as a whole. Second, make an inventory or log of images using categories that reflect and assist research goals. This is a similar process to how many ethnographers take an inventory of various types of field notes. Third, engage in a structured analysis process. Collier writes:

> Go through the evidence with specific questions—measure distance, count, compare. The statistical information may be plotted on graphs, listed in tables, or entered into a computer for statistical analysis. Produce detailed descriptions. (p. 39)

Fourth, search for meaning and draw conclusions based on the entire visual record. Collier also suggests creating an annotation key to allow for comparative analysis (p. 51), team analysis (p. 54), and photo maps (pp. 54–55).

Many of the practices pertaining to anthropological uses of photography have influenced the expansive field of visual research. The analysis procedures suggested by Collier have informed, for example, visual content analysis (which is not reviewed in this book).

- How can social researchers include visual art in their research practices?

The visual arts–based methods researchers have created offer several options, including using art that exists independent of the research in order to study something that it articulates or questions it poses about social life; having research participants create art in order to express or get at some aspect of their lives that would otherwise remain untapped; creating visual models in order to assist data analysis and interpretation; and creating art as a part of the representation of data.

Visual Art as Data and Methodological Intervention: Identity Struggles and Social Power

As a pervasive social product visual art is a significant source of information about the social world, including cultural aspects of social life; economic and political structures; identity issues at the global, national, group, and individual levels; and many other issues. Given the vast range of social phenomena to which art can speak, in this section I focus primarily on how visual art can be used with respect to diverse identity issues, which includes the cultural, representational, economic, and political dimensions of identity. Within these uses of art in the social sciences there are multiple methodologies for accessing subjugated voices long prohibited from participating in collective historical representation.

- How can visual art reify or challenge stereotypes?
- How can visual art serve as a method of exposing and altering unequal relations of power, privilege, and oppression?

Visual Art as a Method of "Aesthetic Intervention"

bell hooks has been at the forefront of theorizing about the relationship between visual art and group identity struggles, paying great attention to the macro contexts in which these struggles over representation occur. Although her work is largely theoretical, and it is that aspect of her work that must first be addressed, there are methodological implications to her analysis.

In *Art on My Mind: Visual Politics* (1995) hooks conceptualizes art as a medium for conveying political ideas, concepts, beliefs, and other information about the culture in which it was produced, including dominant views of race, class, and gender. Furthermore, informed by her engaged feminist politics, hooks makes a persuasive case that race, class, and gender shape who makes art, who sells it, what is sold, who values it, how it is valued, who writes about it, and how it is written about. In this respect art can function as a site of exclusion. However, for hooks, visual art also carries a transformative power that can resist and dislodge stereotypical ways of thinking.

Visual art is therefore an important medium through which struggles over representation occur. The use of visual art in social research may therefore appeal to researchers working from feminist, postcolonial, and other critical perspectives. bell hooks writes: "Representation is a crucial location of struggle for any exploited and oppressed people asserting subjectivity and decolonization of the mind" (1995, p. 3). In hooks's framework, art can serve two primary functions with respect to group representation: (1) recognition of the familiar and (2) defamiliarization. In terms of the former, visual art can depict aspects of how social life really is for people differentially located in the social order, or how life can be imagined.

In addition, not all groups are represented in art. This underrepresentation occurs in two ways. First, many groups who are underrepresented in art cannot turn to (legitimized) paintings, for example, to see representations that they can identify with. In this respect, hooks notes that in black culture there is very little opportunity for people to recognize "self" in art. Second, there are gross distortions and stereotypical characterizations in artistic representation, with some groups systematically privileged over others. Thus visual art can foster stereotypical ways of thinking. In terms of the latter—that is, the capacity of art to promote defamiliarization—visual art can propel people to look at something in a new way, which is critical to social change. In this respect, visual art can transgress racist and sexist ideologies and has a resistive and transformational capability. Visual art can jar people into *seeing* something differently. This kind of consciousness-raising, unleashed by images, may not be possible in textual form. In this regard, painter Edward Hopper once said, "If you could say it in words there would be no reason to paint."

hooks offers a methodological strategy of "aesthetic intervention" for researching this aspect of artistic practice. Specifically, she analyzes the work of artist Emma Amos, who represented people and the political cultural context in which they operate. For hooks, Amos's work harnesses the power of visual images and their cultural symbolism to reimagine shared (collective) images in a new context and correspondingly jolt people into seeing differently. For example, destructive historical images of the Ku Klux Klan can be used in contemporary art in order to expose their dangerous historical uses, raise awareness and social consciousness, and foster social change. Therefore, this kind of artistic "intervention" that unleashes the *oppositional potential* of art is consistent with feminist and other critical epistemologies that have a strong interest in social justice. The increased awareness and heightened feminist consciousness this method cultivates are necessary preconditions for any grassroots social change. How does visual culture contribute to group identity?

- What methods are available for studying visual culture as a site of social struggle?
- How can researchers use the visual arts for studying race, class, gender, and sexuality?

Visual Cultural Archaeology and Subjugated Perspectives

The potential for visual art to reveal subjugated perspectives and intervene in historically oppressive processes of representation is central to Rolling's (2005) research, in which he investigates how images in visual culture contribute to a person's identity, focusing particularly on the African American experience as "other." As a site where struggles over identity and representation are played out, visual culture is a space of contention where ideas of normalcy are created, and out of which the idea of the "other" emerges. From this theoretical vantage point Rolling proposes "visual cultural archaeology" as a method for accessing the insidious ways in which visual culture creates images of normalcy and otherness. Rolling writes:

> Visual cultural archeology reveals that there is a grid of socially constructed narratives that together constitute what becomes "socially visible" as an acceptable identity, as a range of credible reinterpretations of a normalized identity, and as a range of visual shortcomings inhabiting social acceptability. (p. 23)

This method, grounded in critical theoretical perspectives, can be applied to suit the research interests of those studying the representation of sexuality, gender, and any number of contested social identities, as well as their interlocking nature. This approach enables a researcher to qualitatively investigate the relationship between visual culture and changing relations of dominance and oppression.

Similar to Rolling's research on images and racial identity, Susan Finley (2002) conducted extensive research about imagery and gender identity. She was ultimately interested in engaging in a dialogue with teachers regarding the ways they may or may not unintentionally model media-defined gender roles for their students. Her research used images from the mass media as the raw material for her artistic investigation. Finley studied media images and the impact that they have on young women's self-image, and in this way she both studied visual images and used visual art as a means of soliciting further data.

First, Finley conducted a traditional feminist qualitative analysis of media images portraying females. She then categorized the data into possible identities that women may develop from the cumulative impact of the images. Out of these identity categories Finley (2002) constructed 12 panels of collages depicting women's roles, thus creating new art out of the visual images. Conscious of how the media images she selected could reify stereotypes about women she took measures to counteract that risk. She emphasized discordant images and arranged the images in such a way as to promote a sense that "image was being 'played' with in mischievous ways" (p. 174).

In this project Finley viewed the female body as the location of both inquiry and emancipation (2002, p. 166):

> I rewrite those cultural metaphors through the concrete language of the body rendered in the symbolic forms of collage. The collages (both literally and figuratively) tear apart the bodies of women, and then reconstruct

those metaphors in ways that make it difficult to ignore the constructions of female bodies or to ignore the meanings that we habitually attach to those constructions. (p. 167)

With the goal of creating awareness regarding their role as gender models and contributing to a project of critical pedagogy, she presented the collages to teachers. The collages served as a point of departure for a dialogue about images and women's roles. Finley inquired as to whether the teachers embodied any of these conventional roles in class and learned that they did. Among her conclusions, she posited that socially constructed media images are unconsciously adopted by teachers and help model female roles for young women—roles that are therefore limited and socially constructed. Methodologically her project would not have been possible without the creation of visual art—in this case, collages.

- What techniques are available for implementing collage as a research method?

Collage as a Method

Collage combines our everyday reality—bits of photographs, newspaper, found objects from everyday life—with paint or ink, thus merging the illusionary with the actual, art with society, aesthetics with everyday/every night life. (Diaz, 2002, p. 148)

Collage is a particular visual arts-based research practice. As discussed in the previous section, collage was an integral component of Finley's research on media images and the modeling of female gender roles. Vaughan (2004) used the collage method to create new meanings out of selected images. She views collage as a method of gathering, selecting, analysis, synthesis, and presentation—a process that is strikingly similar to more traditional qualitative research.

Diaz (2002) also uses collage as a research tool. Specifically, Diaz offers a method of "collage with text," which blends images and text in an attempt to create a reality and find meaning. She explains that the textual collage is both a work of art and an information-bearing subject. The *juxtaposition of words and images* opens up new meanings that would not be possible without the incorporation of both text and visual imagery. In this vein, Diaz explains that the visual arts can open up new dialogues among diverse people, provide new insights, enhance reflection, and offer a new way to critique a subject.

Figures 7.1–7.6 are part of a series of collage-style artworks created by fine arts professor Maryjean Viano Crowe. This series is an example of how artist-scholars can employ collage as a method of addressing both macro and micro issues as well as their interrelatedness. The series (1993–1994) is titled *All Consuming Myths* and examines gendered social relations in middle-class white America in the 1950s from the perspective of the artist, who was a girl during that time and watched her mother and other women perform gender roles revolving around the preparation of baked goods (which in the art serve as an actuality, a symbol, and a metaphor). The resulting collages juxtapose images in order to expose new and multiple meanings. The series artfully links the macro context of patriarchal culture in which femininity was scripted and enacted to the personal experience of one girl, now a reflective woman. The artist's statement follows:

Here is my memory ...
I am sitting at the pink Formica kitchen table watching my mother construct a cake for my birthday party. A small vinyl doll with a slightly askew wig and stark eyes that blink open and closed is placed within the hollowed-out center of two round layer cakes piled atop each other, secured with a slathering of frosting. It is sometime in the 1950s and my mother is happy, content at this fanciful task of inventing a doll cake, a dream girl for my delight.

Through the magic of food coloring, my cake evolves. Her vanilla frosting gown, sugary and feminine, is transformed into a palette of colorful swirls, complete with frosting flowerettes. Later, my girlfriends and I will eat this cake, cutting away at her slice by slice, deconstructing her colorful ensemble to literally feast upon her. But for now she is safe, beautiful and insulated within the folds of her confectionary cocoon And I am happy at the kitchen table, watching my mother as she frosts and listening to stories of her girlhood hopes and dreams.

It is sometime in the 1950s, and so I lick the frosting from the bowl, willing to consume the dream.

Mj Viano Crowe

The use of collage and metaphor inform the meanings a viewer can derive from the works. As the artist notes in her statement, the pieces merge her personal subjective experiences as a girl and later a reflective woman with larger macro issues, from a gendered perspective. As with all art there are multiple interpretations.

From a feminist perspective this series visually represents a range of urgent social issues. For example, there is a commentary about women's roles as homemakers, as evidenced in "Pie in the Sky." The relationship between women's homemaking, embodied in baking, and the standard heterosexual romance scripts that may help structure their fantasy and "real" lives, is perhaps illustrated in "The Bake-Off." This piece speaks to larger issues about how women's relationships (with men, with other

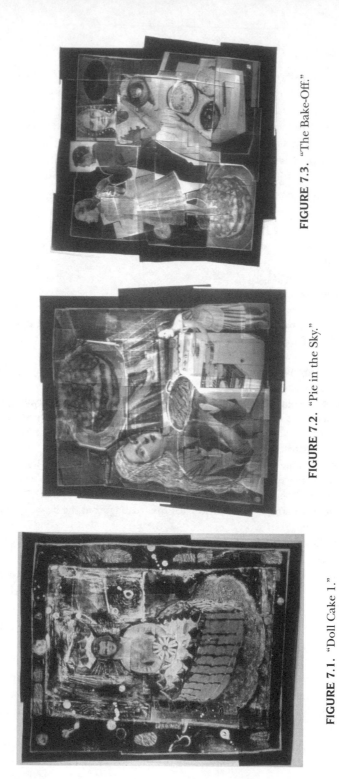

FIGURE 7.3. "The Bake-Off."

FIGURE 7.2. "Pie in the Sky."

FIGURE 7.1. "Doll Cake 1."

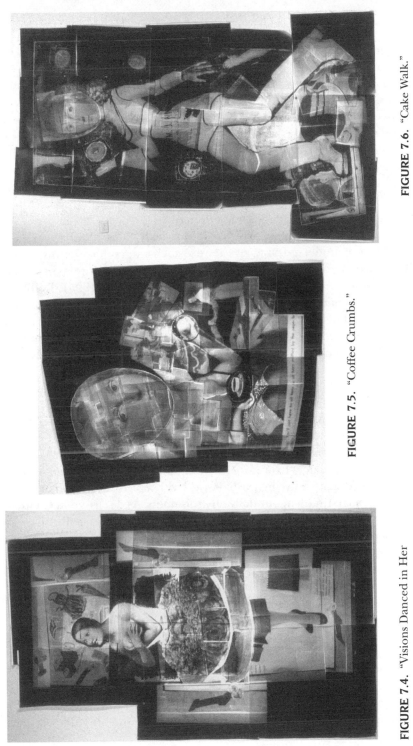

FIGURE 7.6. "Cake Walk."

FIGURE 7.5. "Coffee Crumbs."

FIGURE 7.4. "Visions Danced in Her Head."

225

women, and with themselves) are structured in a patriarchal society. "Visions Danced in Her Head" and "Doll Cake" link the metaphor of baked goods to female body image, beauty, and independence, among many other issues. The multiple meanings addressed in the pieces allow the dynamic nature of society to emerge as well. For example, "Coffee Crumbs" and "Cake Walk" use the same collage style and food metaphor to explore women's changing roles in society, the merging of the public and private spheres, the pressures on women to balance and negotiate their changing roles, and many other social issues. What is most important when examining this series is that meanings are not closed off, but rather open, multiple, suggested, and implied.

As seen in the original artwork of Maryjean Viano Crowe, visual art can alter our understanding of identity, such as gender identity, while also speaking to the larger dynamic sociohistorical context in which our evolving identities develop. Furthermore, hooks's (1995), Rolling's (2005), and Finley's (2002) research all contributes greatly to our understanding of how visual art influences group identity in powerful and complicated ways, including how identity develops in a dynamic context propelled by sociohistorical forces.

Visual Phenomenology

Whatever "human nature" may be, it is no doubt social. As feminist scholar Judith Lorber (1994) famously explains, the paradox of human nature is that it is necessarily social. Therefore human experiences cannot be understood separately from the environments in which they occur. It is well accepted that we live in a visual world with a historically specific multitude of visual stimuli in our daily environments. As discussed in Chapter 4 with respect to music and the penetrating effect of sound—also an inextricable and significant part of modern human experience—when our normative environment becomes highly visual then the visual becomes a part of how our consciousness develops. It is in this context that Noe (2000) suggests merging art and the study of perceptual consciousness.

Specifically, Noe (2000) proposes that art can be an effective, although previously neglected, tool for phenomenological research (a perspective that places experience at the center of knowledge-building). In this regard, he writes, "To describe experience *is* to describe the experienced world" (p. 125). The implication of Noe's work is that if researchers working from a phenomenology framework are interested in accessing experience, and experience now occurs within a visual landscape, experience is embedded within its visual context. Noe proposes that phenomenologists refine their "conception of experience as a mode of interactive engagement with the environment" (p. 124) and therefore offers visual phenomenology as a method for investigating visual experience.

Similarly, Saarnivaara (2003) explores the transgressive experience of art from a phenomenological perspective that emphasizes experience and description. She ultimately shows how this approach illustrates "the enslaving effects of convention" (p. 582) that stem from traditional research practices that falsely polarize inquiry and art (the former as conceptual and the latter as experiential) (p. 582). The merging of art and phenomenology has implications for sociologists working from this theoretical framework and as a result we may continue to see increases in visual sociology.

Visual Arts-Based Participatory Methods

In one sense, visual arts-based methods are necessarily participatory— that is, visual art has an audience who experiences it. In this regard, Blumenfeld-Jones (2002) notes that the art–research connection is grand because the beauty of art is that it is interpretive and therefore different perceivers will have different interpretations; researchers can learn from these multiple interpretations.

With that said, *visual arts-based participatory methods* are a specific set of practices for incorporating visual art into the research process. Most often these strategies involve research participants creating art that ultimately serves both *as* data, and may also *represent* data. These methods are frequently part of multimethod research designs. It is appropriate to use visual imagery when traditional methods cannot fully access what the researcher is after, and so these tools are sometimes employed after traditional qualitative interviews or ethnography in order to elaborate on the data. This kind of approach may also serve as the point of departure for dialogue (in the form of interviews and the like), in that case coming at the beginning of a multimethod research design. *Photo elicitation* is at times used in interview projects. This method relies on using photographs as prompts to "unlock" or dislodge knowledge (Holm, 2008).

When considering participatory visual arts-based methods the issue of aesthetics becomes important. Despite the potential for visual art to captivate and impress messages upon viewers, when amateurs are invited into the art-making process, certainly they cannot be expected to possess artistic ability or training. Therefore, in participatory projects the aesthetic quality of the resulting visual art takes a back seat to the other advantages of the methodology. Moreover, although produced by amateurs, the visual art produced by research participants can still be quite powerful with respect to conveying emotion and the multiple meanings articulated via the art.

- How can visual arts-based participatory methods access hidden dimensions of social life? What can these methods reveal that other methods cannot?
- How can these methods help researchers link the micro level of experience with the macro level of sociohistorical and symbolic context?

Visual Arts-Based Participatory Methods, Social Context, and Education

Knowles and Thomas (2002) conducted empirical research using a visual arts-based participatory method. Their study revolved around an exploration of place and sense of place in school (p. 122) and was therefore about people's subjective experiences in a particular kind of institutionalized social setting. This topic invites individual narratives as well as emergent patterns across the data. Knowles and Thomas asked a sample of students to use art in order to convey how they see themselves and what they think about school as a place to be. They requested that students apply a "model of structure to their inquiry and artistry" and supplied them with seven multimedium elements: self-portrait, memory map, photo of place, narrative, photo of self in place, found object, and two- or three-dimensional artwork (p. 125). Students were also able to textually describe and explain their art. In this way, the art can be viewed as both the method of inquiry and a springboard for more conventional qualitative inquiry.

As a result of this artistic participatory method the researchers learned a great deal about students' feelings, their struggles, and their challenges with respect to "fitting in" at school. For example, one student created a self-portrait that she explained in this way: "My portrait is cropped closely around my face to represent the lack of freedom I feel at school" (p. 127). Knowles and Thomas (2002) reflect that their arts-based approach allowed them to gain a greater understanding than traditional qualitative interviews would have.

Moreover, visual arts-based methods allow for "synergistic practices" that foster a holistic view of the research project, where there is a tight fit between the research goals and the methods employed. Arguably, the creative process and verbal follow-up could be an empowering experience for the research participants as well, where they retain control, share their experiences, and have their feelings and perspective taken seriously (which is a form of validation). Knowles and Thomas (2002) reach the following conclusions regarding their methodology:

> By immersing ourselves in their art, we focused on the depictions of place and the feelings evoked; the drama, mood, and tone of the images; the interrelatedness and coherence of the images with the text; the emphasis given to place and theme in the work as a whole; the balance and composition of the images; and the relationship between the images, text and maps. (p. 126)

Knowles and Thomas found an arts-based participatory method very effective in their study of subjective experiences within a specific social setting.

Kim Hershorn (2005) used a visual arts-based participatory method in order to explore how students in urban school settings feel about violence in their environments. The visual arts were initially chosen as a research tool because this form of art has the capacity to highlight differences and commonalities and to promote dialogue and problem-solving. Hershorn conducted arts-based workshops in which students were specifically asked to draw or otherwise create a picture that depicted "violence and destructive behavior *from their own lives*" (p. 2, original emphasis). Despite the instructions, many of the students incorporated media images of "war and bloodshed" into their visual art (pp. 2–3). This significant result would not have been possible without the use of a participatory arts-based method as the students' visual art, *not their verbal communication*, exposed this important trend.

Hershorn theorized that these results indicate how global crises affect young people's psyches in significant ways. As a result of these findings, which make a powerful link between the individual and the media with respect to violence (or the micro and macro, private and public), Hershorn went on to another phase of the research project focusing on the media coverage of the Iraq War and 9/11 and its effect on the individual. She ultimately concluded that citizens are only exposed to some images of war (and 9/11), those that are particularly gruesome and serve to terrorize, as opposed to the more hopeful, inspirational images to emerge out of these tragic events. Hershorn proposed that the public needs to become more visually literate (a protective measure), and artistic exploration is a means of accomplishing this. In this study, the participant creation of visual art opened the research up in these new ways.

Technology-Based Visual Arts Methods

Cameras provided early visual anthropologists with a new research tool—they allowed researchers to see social reality differently, ask different questions, and represent research findings in new ways. Recent technological developments have again had a major impact on visual methodologies. Holm (2008) notes that contemporary innovations include CD-ROMs, home photo-printing, and "photoblogs" (which can be analyzed as diaries that are housed on the Web). To this list I would add PhotoShop as a tool that is employed by social researchers. *Video diaries* are also increasingly common, according to Holm. Ruby (2005) posits that digital interactive ethnographies are the latest innovation in visual anthropology (as cited in Holm, 2008).

Photovoice as a Social Action Research Method

Photovoice has rapidly become a popular research method in public health research (Holm, 2008). This method relies on giving research participants cameras so that they can take photographs that can be used to advocate for community improvement (see Berg, 2007; Holm, 2008). Holm (2008) suggests that the practice of this method can be grounded in critical consciousness-raising theories. Wang (2005) suggests the following stages in photovoice research (see *www.photovoice.com/method/index.html*):

> Conceptualizing the problem; defining broader goals and objectives; recruiting policymakers as the audience for photovoice findings; training the trainers; conducting photovoice training; devising the initial theme/s for taking pictures; taking pictures; facilitating group discussion; critical reflection and dialogue; selecting photographs for discussion; contextualizing and storytelling; codifying issues, themes, and theories; documenting the stories; conducting the formative evaluation; reaching policymakers, donors, media, researchers, and others who may be mobilized to create change. (quoted in Holm, 2008, p. 330)

It will be interesting to see how changes in the technological landscape continue to influence these practices. For example, to what extent will technological ability and not artistic ability per se affect the aesthetics of these methodological practices? Furthermore, how will ethical issues such as confidentiality be dealt with?

- How can visual art be used to create meanings?
- How can the visual arts be used as analytical and interpretive tools?
- How can the visual arts be used as a representational form? What issues need to be considered when representing textual data in visual form?

Data Analysis, Interpretation, and Representation

Visual art is often thought of as a potential source of data or as a creative means of representation. However, the usefulness of visual art extends into the realm of analysis and interpretation, key components of the research endeavor. In fact, one of the major strengths of using visual methods of analysis and interpretation is that they call attention to the interpretive phase of research, which, due to conventions and practical constraints, is often rushed. In addition, the visual representation of data, as already discussed throughout this chapter, opens up a space for multiple interpretations and perspectives. There are many different ways that the visual can be incorporated into both the analysis and representation phases of social research in service of the researcher's agenda; the following examples are meant to serve as illustrations of some available techniques, although there are many others as well.

Maps, Models, and Diagrams

Visual art techniques are now being used in methodological approaches to interpretation. The process of conducting research is always a meaning-making activity, and explicitly so in qualitative research. Whether conducted within a paradigm based on "discovering" and "revealing" meaning, or one that posits the "creation" and the "construction" of meaning(s), social research is about generating meaning from data. Therefore, the process of analysis and interpretation is vital to the research endeavor.

Despite the inseparable nature of analysis to knowledge, analysis and interpretation are often hurried or not fully disclosed in the final work. This is particularly problematic in qualitative research, which is purported to be an inductive and holistic process, often with interpretation woven into the entire process via grounded theory and other strategies. Hunter, Lusardi, Zucker, Jacelon, and Chandler (2002) collaborated to discuss the process of making meaning in qualitative health care research, reviewing how various arts-based methods aided what they deem the "incubation phase" in which ideas percolate, patterns emerge, and original conclusions develop (p. 389). They refer to this vital period as "intellectual chaos"; however, they are quick to note techniques available for structuring this activity (p. 389).

With respect to visual analysis, Donna Zucker, one of the five health care researchers, employed maps or models as a means of allowing her information and data to become visual so that she might *see* it differently during multiple interpretive moments. In addition to maps and models, diagrams also serve as a similar heuristic device. Zucker self-identifies as a visual learner and consequently the visual representation of her data fostered heightened idea generation. Zucker created visual maps during three phases of her project. The first map was linked to her immersion in existing scholarship and was made during her contemplations of the literature review. The second map was constructed during data collection and the last during coding and analysis (although clearly analysis and interpretation were ongoing parts of her research). This strategy deepened the "incubation phase," allowed relationships between data to emerge that may otherwise have remained hidden, and weaved interpretation throughout the research design in a systematic and holistic manner that could later be explained and reflected on.

Hybridity and the Third Space: Words into Pictures and Pictures into Words

Throughout this chapter visual data and the visual representation of data have been reviewed, including visual anthropology, the participatory creation of art, the collage method, and mapping/diagramming. To draw near a conclusion it is necessary to consider what it means to transform text-based data into visual imagery. It is this very issue that Sava and Nuutinen (2003) explore in their collaborative research that seeks to create a dialogue between inquiry and art. Specifically, they empirically and theoretically examine the hybrid or "third space" created as art and inquiry, or image and word meet, which they view as a merging of the subjective and objective.

For their project Sava served as the researcher-writer who created the words and Nuutinen functioned as the artist who created the images. This was a three-tier project consisting of (1) the word–picture performance, (2) reflective textual dialogue, and (3) a general discussion about the word–picture performance and reflections on it. The project involved the production of seven textual messages and seven drawings that were not paired together simultaneously until a panel discussion. In addition to invited audience discussion that allowed the "reader" to engage in meaning-making, the writer and artist each wrote their reflections independent of one another. They had previously agreed to allow for ample freedom of "inner voice" while remaining attentive to the main theme of "the dialogue between word and picture, between inquiry and art" (2003, p. 516). Sava and Nuutinen's research suggests several things about the relationship between text and visual art:

> First, in the performative dialogue between writer and maker of pictures, it can be a question of *change, transformation of word/text into a picture* (or *vice versa*), *of sliding, flowing, streaming*, perhaps also a question of *translation from one language to another*. Second, texts and pictures can form an *intertextual surface, an associative texture*. Third, pictures can function rather as *illustrations of the text*, or in the opposite process, *text as illustrator of the pictures*, or they form a mutual, living dialogue, a unified story or dialogical state. (p. 532, original emphasis)

As alluded to in the last point, this research contributes to ongoing scholarship in the area of hybridity (rapidly increasing with globalization, as discussed in Chapter 4 on music). Sava and Nuutinen note that the "third space"

> is strongly experiential, sensory, multi-interpretive, like a fleeting shadow, intuitive and ever changing ... must accept borderline existence of the two or more worlds, the meeting place as a *mixed stream of fluids*, as something multi-layered, not known, always to be created anew, as the field of many understandings. (p. 532, original emphasis)

This exploratory collaborative project contributes to scholarship in multiple areas while raising significant questions about what occurs when researchers translate words into pictures or pictures into words, and how audiences perceive the relationships between words and images.

Checklist of Considerations

✓ How does the use of visual art help address the issues in this study? What alternatives are available and why is visual art most appropriate in this study? How does the theoretical framework support the use of a visual approach?

✓ Will the visual art in this study exist independent of the research project or be created via participatory methods or be created as a representational form, and if so, by whom? How will the visual art component speak to the other components in multimethod research?

✓ What method best suits my research objectives (e.g., photography, collage, visual archeology, participatory methods)?

✓ How will visual art be used (e.g., data collection, analysis, interpretation, representation)? If there is a transfer between words and images, how will this "translation process" be understood? How will authenticity be evaluated?

Conclusion

Visual analysis is an expansive topic; however, this chapter is meant to serve as an introduction to some of the theoretical and methodological issues at the intersection of the visual arts and social research. In the following article Carolyn Jongeward describes using visual portraits in a research project about how adults connect to their creativity. Jongeward reviews the contribution of visual portraits in this project and also the larger relationship between artistic inquiry and social inquiry, arguing that the qualitative paradigm is enriched via the nature of visual research. Moreover, Jongeward speaks to the unique power of "the image" with respect to making and evoking meaning.

DISCUSSION QUESTIONS AND ACTIVITIES

1. How can visual art be used to reinforce or challenge stereotypes? How can visual art be employed in a research project aimed at accessing subjugated perspectives? What is "visual archaeology"?

2. How can participatory arts-based methods access hidden dimensions of social life? Can other methods accomplish this? What are the differences?

3. How is collage used as a research method? Why might a researcher employ this technique?

4. What can visual art reveal about the mind–body connection? How can art help bridge this connection within social research? What is "visual phenomenology"?

5. How can the visual arts be used during analysis and interpretation?

6. Collect a small sample of visual images from a magazine or newspaper. Without context, what stories do the images tell? What meanings are communicated? Create a collage out of the images considering the role of juxtaposition in meaning-making. Now what meanings are communicated?

SUGGESTED READINGS

Collier, J., Jr., & Collier, M. (1996). *Visual anthropology: Photography as a research method.* Albuquerque: University of New Mexico Press. (Original work published 1986)

This classic text on visual anthropology is a must-read for anyone interested in photography as a research method, although the book is also relevant for those interested in visual analysis more broadly. Original research examples help illustrate the points throughout the text.

Emmison, M., & Smith, P. (2000). *Researching the visual: Images, objects, contexts and interactions in social and cultural inquiry.* Thousand Oaks, CA: Sage.

This qualitative visual research primer covers a range of topics pertaining to conducting research with visual data. The authors also provide exercises throughout the text suitable for students or researchers who wish to try out some of the techniques in the book.

hooks, b. (1995). *Art on my mind: Visual politics.* New York: The New Press.

In this book, hooks regards art as a method of conveying political ideas, concepts, beliefs, and other information about the culture in which it was produced. In particular, hooks critically examines the relationship between art and interlocking identity categories such as race and gender.

Sullivan, G. (2005). *Art practice as research: Inquiry in the visual arts.* Thousand Oaks, CA: Sage.

This book explores the visual arts as a place of social inquiry, covering both theoretical and methodological advancements at the intersection of art and inquiry. This book is quite sophisticated and appropriate for advanced readers.

van Leeuwen, T., & Jewitt, C. (Eds.). (2001). *Handbook of visual analysis.* Thousand Oaks, CA: Sage.

This edited collection provides nine chapters covering a range of perspectives on visual analysis, as well as methodological practices. Topics covered include content analysis, visual anthropology, cultural studies, semiotics, psychoanalysis, iconography, film, and ethnomethodology.

SUGGESTED WEBSITES AND JOURNALS

Arts and Humanities in Higher Education: An International Journal of Theory, Research and Practice
ahh.sagepub.com

This peer-reviewed journal publishes articles and reviews based on scholarship in the arts and humanities in higher education. The journal has an international outlook and is useful for teachers as well as researchers.

ArtsJournal
   www.artsjournal.com/visual.shtml

   ArtsJournal was founded in 1999 and features daily links to stories taken from more than 200 English-language newspapers, magazines, and publications featuring writing about arts and culture. Stories from sites that charge for access are excluded. This is an excellent resource for articles and to other venues that deal with art and culture.

International Journal of Education through Art
   www.intellectbooks.co.uk/journals.appx.php?issn=17435234

   Published three times a year, the *International Journal of Education through Art* is an interdisciplinary journal that promotes relationships between art and education. Particular emphasis is placed on articles and visual materials that critically reflect on the relationship between education and art; propose original ways of rethinking the status of education and art education; address the role of teaching and learning in either formal or informal educational contexts and alongside issues of age, gender, and social background; adopt an open and inventive interpretation of research-based analysis; and promote and experiment with visual/textual forms of representing art education activities, issues, and research.

Visual Studies
   www.visualsociology.org/publications.html

   Published three times a year by the International Visual Sociology Association, this multidisciplinary peer-reviewed journal publishes "visually oriented" articles that represent empirical visual research, studies of visual and material culture, visual research methods, and visual means of communicating about the social and cultural world.

Journal of Visual Arts Practice
   www.ovid.com/site/catalog/Journal/2444.jsp?top=2&mid=3&bottom=7&subsection=12

   This journal addresses issues of contemporary content and practice in fine-arts studios. Over the past decades fine-arts practices have expanded from the traditional media of painting, sculpture, and printmaking to include installation, performance, film, video, and digitized media.

Art Journal
   www.collegeart.org/artjournal

   Founded in 1941, this peer-reviewed journal aims to provide a forum for scholarship and visual exploration in the visual arts; to operate in the spaces between commercial publishing, academic presses, and artist presses; to be pedagogically useful; to explore relationships among diverse forms of art practice and production, as well as among art making, art history, visual studies, theory, and criticism; to give artists, art historians, and other writers in the arts a publishing venue; to be responsive to current issues in the arts, both nationally and globally; and to focus on topics related to 20th- and 21st-century concerns.

Oxford Art Journal
oaj.oxfordjournals.org

The *Oxford Art Journal* is a peer-reviewed journal that publishes innovative critical work in art history. It is committed to the political analysis of visual art and material representation from a variety of theoretical perspectives, and has carried work covering themes from antiquity to contemporary art practice. The journal also publishes extended reviews of major contributions to the field.

Technoetic Arts: A Journal of Speculative Research
www.ovid.com/site/catalog/Journal/2453.jsp?top=2&mid=3&bottom=7&subse ction=12

This peer-reviewed journal publishes work dealing with cutting-edge ideas, projects, and practices arising from the confluence of art, science, technology, and consciousness research.

International Visual Sociology Association (IVSA)
www.visualsociology.org

The purpose of the IVSA is to promote the study, production, and use of visual images, data, and materials in teaching, research, and applied activities, and to foster the development and use of still photographs, film, video, and electronically transmitted images in sociology and other social sciences and related disciplines and applications.

REFERENCES

Berg, B. (2007). *Qualitative research methods for the social sciences.* New York: Pearson.

Blumenfeld-Jones, D. S. (2002). If I could have said it, I would have. In C. Bagley & M. B. Cancienne (Eds.), *Dancing the data* (pp. 90–104). New York: Peter Lang.

Collier, J., Jr., & Collier, M. (1996). *Visual anthropology: Photography as a research method.* Albuquerque: University of New Mexico Press. (Original work published 1986)

Collier, M. (2001). Approaches to analysis in visual anthropology. In T. van Leeuwen & C. Jewitt (Eds.), *Handbook of visual analysis* (pp. 35–60). London: Sage.

Diaz, G. (2002). Artistic inquiry: On Lighthouse Hill. In C. Bagley & M. B. Cancienne (Eds.), *Dancing the data* (pp. 147–161). New York: Peter Lang.

Finley, S. (2002). Women myths: Teacher self-images and socialization to feminine stereotypes. In C. Bagley & M. B. Cancienne (Eds.), *Dancing the data* (pp. 162–176). New York: Peter Lang.

Fitzhenry, R. I. (Ed.). (1993). *The Harper book of quotations* (3rd ed.). New York: HarperPerennial.

Hershorn, K. (2005, May). *Learning through arts-based action research: Creative approaches to destructive dynamics in our schools and in our world.* Paper presented at the International Congress of Qualitative Inquiry, Urbana–Champaign, IL.

Hesse-Biber, S. N. (1996). *Am I thin enough yet?: The cult of thinness and the commercialization of identity.* New York: Oxford University Press.

Hockings, P. (Ed.). (2003). *Principles of visual anthropology.* New York: de Gruyter.

Holm, G. (2008). Visual research methods: Where are we and where are we going? In S. N. Hesse-Biber & P. Leavy (Eds.), *Handbook of emergent methods* (pp. 325–342). New York: Guilford Press.

hooks, b. (1995). In our glory: Photography and black life. In b. hooks (Ed.), *Art on my mind: Visual politics* (pp. 54–64). New York: New Press.

Hunter, H., Lusardi, P., Zucker, D., Jacelon, C., & Chandler, G. (2002). Making meaning: The creative component in qualitative research. *Qualitative Health Research Journal, 12*(3), 388–398.

Knowles, J. G., & Thomas, S. M. (2002). Artistry, inquiry, and sense-of-place: Secondary school students portrayed in context. In C. Bagley & M. B. Cancienne (Eds.), *Dancing the data* (pp. 121–132). New York: Peter Lang.

Lorber, J. (1994). *Paradoxes of gender.* New Haven, CT: Yale University Press.

Mills, G. (1957). Art: An introduction to qualitative anthropology. *Journal of Aesthetics and Art Criticism, 16*(1), 1–17.

Noe, A. (2000). Experience and experiment in art. *Journal of Consciousness Studies, 7*(8–9), 123–135.

Rolling, J. H., Jr. (2005). Visual culture archaeology: A criti/polit:/cal methodology of image and identity. *Cultural Studies ↔ Critical Methodologies, 7*(1), 3–25.

Ruby, J. (2005). The last 20 years of visual anthropology—a critical review. *Visual Studies, 20*(2), 159–170.

Saarnivaara, M. (2003). Art as inquiry: The autopsy of an [art] experience. *Qualitative Inquiry, 9*(4), 580–602.

Sava, I., & Nuutinen, K. (2003). At the meeting place of word and picture: Between art and inquiry. *Qualitative Inquiry, 9*(4), 515–534.

Sprague, J., & Zimmerman, M. (1993). Overcoming dualisms: A feminist agenda for sociological method. In P. England (Ed.), *Theory on gender/feminism on theory* (pp. 255–279). New York: DeGruyter.

Vaughan, K. (2004). Pieced together: Collage as an artist's method for interdisciplinary research. *Journal of Qualitative Methods, 4*(1), 1–21.

Wang, C. (2005). Photovoice: Social change through photography. Available at *www.photovoice.com/method/index.html*

Warren, B. (Ed.). (1993). *Using the creative arts in therapy: A practical introduction.* New York: Routledge.

Visual Portraits
*Integrating Artistic Process
into Qualitative Research*

Carolyn Jongeward

Traditional forms of research limit the nature of research inquiry, interpretation, and representation. In contrast, what would educational research look like if the rigors and sensibilities of artistic practice were valued and visible? I have found that artistic attributes such as aesthetic perception, openness to unknowns, and intuitions of complex wholeness do enhance educational research.

In this article I exemplify research that is informed by artistic practice. I describe how I made visual portraits to represent the uniqueness of each research participant. I explore how artistic ways of knowing and making meaning contribute to qualitative research, and I show the value of making visual images as part of the research process. To appreciate how artistic experience can inform educational research requires an understanding of how making art is both a process of inquiry and a process of creating meaningful forms. Artistic practice is a distinctive activity of research and representation.

Other writers have explored links between qualitative research and artistic experience, for example, Eisner (1991, 1993) and Finley and Knowles (1995). Using the concepts of researcher as artist and artist as researcher, these authors affirm the potential of artistic forms of research representation. By doing so, they create a context in which other artist-researchers can articulate the meaning of their own experiences.

Seeking a Fit
between the Researcher and the Research

I have explored processes of creativity for many years as tapestry designer and weaver (Jongeward, 1990). As educator I have facilitated creativity through teaching adults about design and color. In the process, I learned how important it is for adults to connect with their creativity, and at the same time, how difficult this is to do in practice.

As a form of action research, I developed and facilitated a 10-week course entitled "Design: Focus on Creative Process" through the School of Continuing Studies, University of Toronto. My aim was to create conditions for adults to learn about their perspectives, attitudes, and approaches to creativity (Jongeward, 1995).

Researching adult experiences of learning and creativity, I was guided by principles of "reflexivity, responsiveness, and reciprocality" (Hunt, 1992). Self-reflection, visual image making, and dialogue were fundamental components of the course and the research process. I learned about participants' experiences through their writing, imagery, art projects, exchanges in class, and interviews. In direct response to my subject of inquiry and the kind of process participants were engaged in, I decided to extend my methodology for research interpretation and representation to include the making of visual images.

Through experience making visual images and facilitating others' imagery process, I have come to appreciate the expressive and evocative power of images. In one exercise, for example, I ask students to make marks on paper using crayons in a way that expresses their connection with words evocative of strong emotions. The personal images that emerge are unique. Everyone has a particular quality of experience associated with such emotions as sadness, joy, anger, fear, and peacefulness, and these qualitative differences are evident in the distinctive use of color, shape, and line that forms each image.

During the research process I made visual images at critical times to gain energy, clarity, and insight. While doing data analysis, I created six visual portraits to convey the integrity and diversity of my participants' experiences. Making the portraits was significant both as a methodology for interpretation and representation and also as a means to maintain my own connection with artistic intuitive ways of knowing.

Linking Perspectives
on Tacit Knowledge and Visual Imagery

Within the naturalistic paradigm of qualitative research, the knower is inseparable from the known (Lincoln & Guba, 1985). A researcher's sensitivity, empathy with others, and tolerance for ambiguity play an important part in the process and outcomes of research. According to Hunt (1992), a researcher's intentions, perceptions, and actions must be included in the research process because they are the "most powerful and sensitive means for recording and interpreting our research" (p. 116).

It follows that an educational researcher, as "human instrument" in the research process, needs to be responsive to tacit dimensions of his/her own and others' experiences. This takes practice: Just as artists hone their skills and aesthetic awareness, so too do researchers develop abilities to observe, attend to details, and discover implicit relationships of parts within the whole.

Tacit knowledge becomes known and expressed through symbolic forms. And, as Courtney (1987) states, "The tacit dimension, when symbolically expressed through a medium, is the domain of the arts in particular" (pp. 41–43). Artists engage in experiential inquiry, finding new ways to explore knowledge and meaning as they create. Visual images provide a way to connect with, represent, and give meaning to inner experiences. As nondiscursive expressions of feeling, images convey previously unknown ideas in symbolic forms that have significance and bring understanding and insight (Langer, 1953).

The process of creating visual imagery probes below the level of the rational mind and reveals what cannot be known from that perspective alone. Unanticipated connections can be discovered as an image creates relationships among diverse elements of form and experience bring these into a new wholeness.

Visual Portraits:
Portraying Richness and Complexity

The idea to create visual portraits as an alternative way of interpreting and representing my research emerged unexpectedly. I was working on data analysis, involved in the demands of categorizing interviews and participants' journal writings. Reading and rereading, comparing and contrasting different aspects of what participants said or wrote, I felt close to their attitudes and perspectives. However, the sustained analytic process of segmenting and coding data made me want to have an image of the whole person.

I decided to work visually to weave together multiple threads of each person's perspectives and approaches to creative process. Calling upon intuitive and visual sensibilities that I knew from experience would help me see a sense of the whole, I explored the richness of participants' experiences by making visual portraits.

Before describing key elements of this process, a note is necessary: Color, line, shape, and rhythmic relationship of parts within the whole contribute a meaningful particularity to any image. The reader of this article cannot see the color subtleties, intensities, contrasts, blending, repetitions, proportions, all integral to the content conveyed.

I started the portraits by focusing on a participant whose passion and struggle to connect with her creativity made a very strong impression on me. Lillian's words and images filled my thoughts. I picked blue and black oil pastels and began to make a circular form. Gradually an image emerged as I intuitively integrated elements that I knew were important in Lillian's experience. I represented her strongly contrasting feelings primarily by creating a dichotomy between the left and right parts of the image. For example, on the left I worked with her favorite colors, blues and reds, which she linked to her emotional nature and feminine sensitivity. On the right I made a plant-like form using yellow, orange, and green, symbolizing the emergence of her direction of personal growth. Lillian rarely used these colors, but she recognized them as representing masculine qualities of intellect and assertion that she felt she needed to develop (see Figure 7.7).

Throughout the process of creating visual portraits for each participant I questioned how to make an image that reflected the integrity and complexity of who they were. As a result, my understanding deepened and my awareness of visual images as a way of making meaning increased. Continually seeking how to express relationships among complex ideas and feelings, I used color and form to capture what I felt to be true to the participant and also to create a unified image. At times, I made "visual quotes" or references, working with materials, techniques, and elements of personal imagery that participants had explored. I also worked with ideas and attitudes that characterized their creative processes.

In one portrait, my guiding idea was the synthesis of a geometric pattern with a spontaneous visual image. This integration of order and randomness let me capture two distinctive yet complementary aspects I saw in Bob, symbolizing the scope of his knowledge and openness. As an aerospace engineer, Bob knew about technical and mathematical aspects

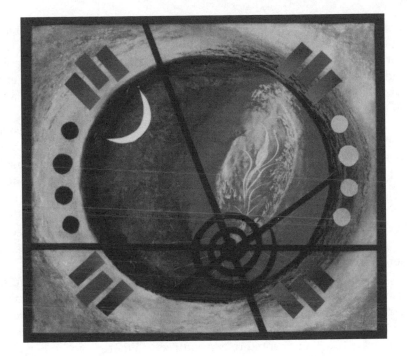

FIGURE 7.7. Visual portrait for Lillian. Oil pastel and cut paper. 11 × 12 inches.

of creativity. However, his primary interest at the time of my work with him was to explore spontaneous imagery and nontechnical aspects of creativity.

Following are stories of three participants and how I worked to convey their perspectives through visual imagery. Marion, an oncology nurse, remembered that ever since she was young she wrote stories, poems, and songs that she sang to herself. As an adult she wanted to be able to write all the time, but she stopped on several occasions, believing she could not write well enough. During the course she began to write again. Through her writing, I discovered a woman with a certain wildness of spirit and longing for freedom and creative expression.

Marion took on a challenging project for herself during the course. She decided to make paper and make a book for her writings. She bought a blender, a book about paper making, and jumped into the process. Discouraged at first because the paper didn't turn out well, she persisted and gradually learned the steps, adjusting her ideas to the needs of the materials. As she made more paper and got better at it, she enjoyed the process.

She began to feel she *could* do something artistic, rather than always feeling that whatever she did would not work. Continuing to write poetry, Marion assembled small handmade paper books using a Japanese bookbinding technique she taught herself. Her last piece of writing at the end of the course intrigued me: "My turtle poem perhaps describes me and my perception of how I was involved in creative process."

I realized that a turtle image would be central to Marion's visual portrait. I began by cutting oval shapes from green tissue paper and combining them in layers with other papers, echoing her own paper and book making. I assembled nine multilayered oval shapes—a central one surrounded by eight smaller ones, like plates on the back of a turtle. At this point I realized the image needed something else. Remembering Marion's metaphor for herself as a place in nature, a fire warm and bright, I placed the green ovals on top of red paper, and the image immediately became more lively.

Initially, the background color was black, but I added turquoise tissue paper, layered over blue construction paper. The black became a narrow border at the end of the image. I recalled a spontaneous image Marion had made in class about her hopes and fears for the future. In that image black represented to Marion everything that got in her way, and blue represented a force of "just doing what really mattered." In her sequence of images, she had pushed the black out to the edges, making more space for the blue. I remembered this description of her imagery simultaneously with my response to the emerging portrait.

From Marion's writing, I selected key statements that represented different stages and perspectives of her experience of learning about herself as creative. The following phrases, which I printed on the top layer of the oval shapes, contain the essence of Marion's story: (a) wanting a way to express myself; (b) having a burning desire to make something; (c) wanting to be proud of what I do; (d) writing, because if I don't I am denying myself; (e) earlier in my life I discounted my creativity—I never even tried because I believed I would fail; (f) wanting to share and not worry about what others will say; (g) convincing myself to do something and getting encouragement to keep trying; (h) learning that something takes practice, frustration, and self-doubt; (i) it's going to be a long process—each day a little more exploration and trying.

Upon finishing this visual portrait, as shown in Figure 7.8, I realized it had a simplicity and childlike quality. The irregularities of torn paper edges resembled the rough edges of Marion's handmade paper. Marion was not concerned with precision, I reminded myself, going against my own tendency for a "finished look."

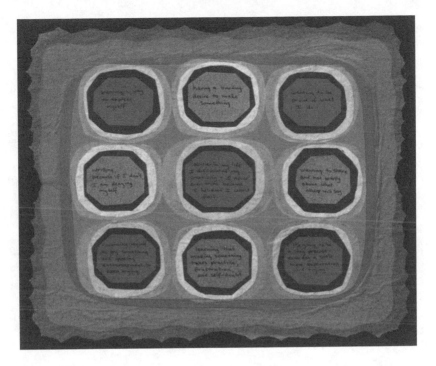

FIGURE 7.8. Visual portrait for Marion. Tissue paper, construction paper, ink. 20½ × 17½ inches.

Jody, a payroll accounts manager, had memories of finger painting as a child. She also remembered coming up with creative ideas for school projects but never feeling she knew how to achieve what she had in mind. She signed up for the creative process course because she wanted to find ways to do things she would gain pleasure from.

Jody felt "behind" others in the class who had already done some kind of artwork. She felt she knew nothing and was just starting out. To begin with, she spent a long time in an art-supply store just looking at materials and deciding what she wanted to do. Eventually she decided to buy a sketchbook and chalk pastels in order to start making images that expressed her feelings while seeing a sunset or a winter landscape in the Rockies. Jody knew she had passion for life, but she didn't let it out. She also knew she didn't have drawing skills, and so she wanted to simply follow her ideas and feelings as they flowed.

While Jody wanted to express her feelings "free-form without thought," she also had many ideas that inhibited her ability to express herself. For her visual portrait, I decided to do a series of spontaneous drawings related to expressions of emotions. This was related to an exercise that Jody had found helped her to get to know herself better.

Color was the medium of choice for capturing and conveying Jody's passion and struggle. I did not plan the images. I explored the feeling behind words that Jody had used to describe her process. I sought to capture the dichotomy and friction between her sense of exploration and constraint. Using chalk pastels on a large piece of paper subdivided into eight sections, I made eight small images. Four images symbolized her expansive, exploratory side, and four symbolized what held her back and stifled her (see Figure 7.9).

Frida did clerical work in a small company that sold business machines. She did not like this work and felt disconnected from herself every day she worked there. She fervently wanted to reconnect with her creativity. When turning 55 she promised herself to do some creative work each day.

As a child in Argentina, Frida had learned many art and craft activities. She was very good at what she did but never received encourage-

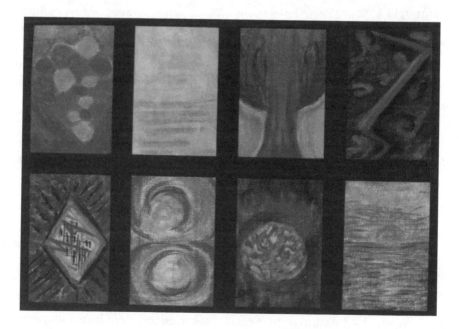

FIGURE 7.9. Visual portrait for Jody. Chalk paste and black paper. 22 × 15 inches.

ment. She never felt valued for who she was. On the contrary, she was often ridiculed for showing her feelings. She learned early on to keep her feelings to herself and never express them.

After moving to Canada and discovering that she was still unhappy, she was helped by a therapist who asked her, "What do you like?" Realizing that she loved color and form, she enrolled at the Ontario College of Art, where she studied for 5 years. However, Frida still did not believe she could ever do anything well enough, and after leaving the art college, she had long gaps between the times of doing creative work.

During the course, Frida worked on highly detailed color pencil drawings of roses. She also showed me collages, especially one she made for her mother who was dying of cancer in Argentina.

In making Frida's portrait, I worked with pencil crayons on a drawing about the size of her small flower drawings. First, I repeated the number five across the bottom of the image, representing the importance of her decision at 55 to commit herself to her creativity. Above the numbers I worked on a section evocative of roots, representing how deeply her creativity was rooted in her life experience.

For the center of the image, I drew a candleholder that emerged from the ground and contained one tall candle and eight red roses. This part of the image was linked directly to the collage Frida had made for her mother: a collage in which Frida said goodbye to her mother, who died before she had completed it.

There are qualities of longing, sadness, and hope in this image. A gray area behind the candlelight represents Frida's sad memories of difficulties as a child, especially relating with her mother. The yellow diamonds are sparks of light. At the top of the image I drew a silver form of a bird in flight, in response to Frida's question, "When is it going to take off?" This question contained her longing to be able to keep a steady continuity of creative effort and expression.

The finished image, as shown in Figure 7.10, has a delicate quality. Frida knew well how to do detailed shading and blending with colored pencils. I experimented and learned throughout the process, but I also tried to keep a lightness of touch and flow of movement while focusing on small details.

Each portrait was different in content, materials, and approach, just as the lives and creative efforts of the participants were highly individual. Creating each portrait brought me new challenges and insights, but most importantly, I felt I lived with an individual's unique way of being and doing while making the portrait. In the end, I created images that embodied my understanding and feeling connection for each person.

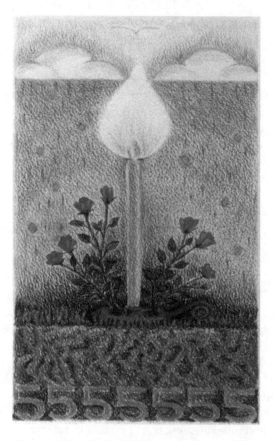

FIGURE 7.10. Visual portrait for Frida. Pencil crayon on paper. 7 × 11 inches.

The Significance of Coherence

When beginning this research, I did not know I would incorporate art-work. I did not set out to do arts-based research. I thought the research process would be very different from what I did as an artist. However, encouraged to begin with myself, my artistic experience and long-standing interest in creativity naturally shaped the research inquiry, interpretation, and representation.

Reflecting on my experience of creating visual portraits, I have identified five major ways in which this artistic process benefited the research as a whole.

1. Integrity of researcher as artist, artist as researcher. It was significant for me to be able to engage in research and simultaneously act

in accord with my values and knowledge from experience. I was able to maintain connection with intuitions, feelings, and visual awareness. My energy was heightened through a creative process of moving toward a truthful image; an image resonant with the particulars of my own and others' experiences.

2. Coherence between visual portraits and the research as a whole. Making visual portraits was coherent with the subject of the research and also the principles of "research as renewal" (Hunt, 1992) that guided my methodology. For example, I not only incorporated similar art materials and processes that participants used during the course, I also mirrored participants' experiences of risk taking by using certain art methods that I had little familiarity with.

3. Intimacy of relatedness between researcher and participants. In making the images I explored and responded to a complex blend of impressions that I experienced in relation to my participants. By seeking to understand their worlds in this way, I felt a depth of connection with each of them.

4. Complementarity of visual portraits and data analysis. Making visual portraits while immersed in the details of research analysis allowed me to balance analytic thought with holistic perception. This way of apprehending subtleties, finding hidden relationships, and seeing the whole involved a shift in mode of thinking and feeling, and the image itself expressed both complexity and unity.

5. Complementarity of visual portraits and participant profiles. Making each portrait was a significant process for discovering and communicating my understanding of participants' experiences. I accompanied each portrait with a written narrative, highlighting and expanding upon key ideas. In this way, visual and verbal representations coincided, giving different perspectives and a larger, more inclusive picture.

Using the metaphor "researcher as artist," Elliot Eisner (1991) has encouraged educational researchers to become more artistic in carrying out their research. While envisioning new approaches to qualitative educational research I believe there is a need to investigate the processes, as well as the forms, of arts-based research. For example: What unique ways of knowing are called upon and developed through artistic processes of investigating, seeing, feeling, being open, integrating, expressing?

An artist seeks to understand something about the world, about self, about materials and ways of making expressive forms. Engaging with materials, thoughts, and feelings, an artist participates in a search. This search to bring something into being requires attention to details, a sense of relatedness among all parts within a whole, and tolerance for the tension of not knowing what will emerge.

Creative process, in all its particularities and contexts, emerges from a coherence between the person creating and what is being created. Stating my view simply, creative process goes something like this:

I work on something (action–interaction).
Something works in me (receptivity–transformation).
Something comes into being (emergent form).
I come to know something (emergent meaning).
Something becomes seen (visibility to others).
I see myself (self-visibility).

Through the practice of creating expressive forms and experiencing a depth of meaning and value in the process, an artist develops and refines affective, intuitive, aesthetic, and relational ways of knowing. Knowledge internalized through experience of engaging in creative process is a key value that an artist can bring to educational research.

Emerging Possibilities for Researchers

Ways of being, knowing, and doing that characterize artistic practice are not exclusive to artists per se. Certain qualities and approaches can be learned and applied by those who want to engage in artistic processes. Researchers can develop their aesthetic awareness, increasing their ability to observe, reflect, and create. This takes practice, but exercising artistic ways of knowing can extend a researcher's capacity to discover and represent meaningful patterns within complex phenomena.

Eisner (1993) wrote, "As sensibility is refined, our ability to construct meaning in a particular domain is refined" (p. 6). For researchers who seek to access tacit dimensions of their own and their participants' experiences, visual image-making offers a unique way of bringing to view and transforming meanings embedded in experiences. Researchers can learn new ways of giving form to ideas, intuitions, and feelings. This process facilitates penetrating to the heart of the matter and gaining insights not possible through rational thought alone.

Integrating artistic processes into educational research is important because this generates unique ways of understanding and representing experiences. Through valuing different ways of perceiving, knowing, and making meaning, an artist-researcher can contribute holistic and intimate perspectives to research. Researcher self-studies of making visual imagery while engaged in educational research is one way to extend knowledge of the potential contribution of arts to qualitative research.

References

Courtney, R. (1987). *The quest: Research and inquiry in arts education.* Lanham, MD: All University Press of America.

Eisner, E. (1991). *The enlightened eye.* New York: Macmillan.

Eisner, E. (1993). Forms of understanding and the future of educational research. *The Educational Researcher, 22*(7), 5–11.

Finley, S., & Knowles, J. G. (1995). Researcher as artist/artist as researcher. *Qualitative Inquiry, 1,* 110–142.

Jongeward, C. (1995). *Connecting with creativity: Adults learning through art making within a supportive group.* Unpublished doctoral dissertation, Ontario Institute for Studies in Education, University of Toronto.

Jongeward, D. (1990). *Weaver of worlds: A women's journey in tapestry.* Rochester, VT: Inner Traditions Press.

Hunt, D. (1992). *The renewal of personal energy.* Toronto: Ontario Institute for Studies in Education Press.

Langer, S. (1953). *Feeling and form: A theory of art.* New York: Scribner.

Lincoln, Y. S., & Guba, E. G. (1985). *Naturalistic inquiry.* Beverly Hills, CA: Sage.

CHAPTER 8

❧

Bridging the Art–Science Divide

The practice seems to yield at least this hard lesson: a story is not
a story until it is told; it is not told until it is heard, it changes—
and becomes open to the beauties and frailties of more change;
or: a story is not a story until it changes.

—DELLA POLLOCK (2006, p. 93)

The story of arts-based research practices is one about fusion, affinity, resonance, and above all *holistic approaches to research* from the point of view of the knowledge-building process and the researcher who is able to merge an artist-scientist identity. The story began at the intersection of social justice movements, theoretical advances, and paradigm expansion. But now it is unfolding in new and exciting directions as the qualitative paradigm shifts and the formerly segregated roles of self, artist, researcher, and teacher are allowed to fuse. As borderlines and borderlands change and even rupture, new spaces for arts-based inquiry emerge.

Method meets art at the intersection of social and political progress, the emergence of alternative theoretical and epistemological groundings, overarching social justice–oriented research initiatives, and the academic shift toward interdisciplinarity and now transdisciplinarity. The merging of the world of science with the world of art has caused a renegotiation of the scientific standards that traditionally guided social scientific research practice while also highlighting the points of convergence between these two formerly disparate worlds. The methodological hybridization that has occurred as a result of these larger shifts, which constitutes the focus of this book, facilitates the objectives many qualitative researchers have long held while simultaneously creating a space where new research questions can be formulated.

Elliot W. Eisner notes that our selection of research topics is inextricably bound to the available knowledge-building tools; he posits that our "capacity to wonder is stimulated" by the kinds of methodological tools and forms of representation with which we are familiar (1997, p. 8). In addition, Eisner suggests that we seek "what we know how to find" (1997, p. 7). These tools shape topic selection, research questions, and research design (from data collection to representation). Sharlene Hesse-Biber and I (2006) suggest that new methods provide ways to "come at things differently." Therefore, methodological innovation is not simply about adding new methods to our arsenal for the sake of "more," but rather opening up new ways to think about knowledge-building: *new ways to see*. Arts-based research practices are about composing, weaving, and orchestrating—creating tapestries of meanings.

Moreover, as noted throughout this volume, sometimes a traditional approach to research is not able to get at, illuminate, or represent what the researcher is interested in. Put simply, sometimes a conventional methodology comes up short. In these instances, methodological innovation might be needed. As reviewed throughout this book, arts-based practices are a significant genre in which innovation is occurring. In this respect, the emergence of an arts-based genre of social research is a part of a larger shift from traditional qualitative practice to the interdisciplinary qualitative paradigm.

The Arts as Research

In everyday social life the arts are often characterized as "universal." Although the arts can be a source of common understanding and serve as a point of convergence (a strength of some arts-based methods), by and large the idea that music or dance serves as a "universal language" is a romanticized view of the arts that fails to consider the larger system in which art is produced and consumed. Art is produced within sociohistorical contexts. There is an institutional context to the production of art, as well as market forces, which together create the value system in which art is legitimized, judged, consumed, and traded. Moreover, philosophical perspectives on art, cultural norms and values, as well as pragmatic concerns also affect the production and consumption of art. Globalization, a multidirectional exchange of cultural artifacts, capital, and technology, also influences artistic production. In this vein, hybrid arts, in both form and content, have been popping up everywhere and can serve as an entrance into significant contemporary questions about cultural exchange/transfer. For these reasons, we may see an increase in arts-based research practices for their compatibility with studies of globalization.

Arguably, the two phenomena that have most propelled the arts into qualitative research practice are the power and immediacy of artistic mediums and the oppositional possibilities of art.

The arts can grab hold of people's attention in powerful ways, making lasting impressions. Art is immediate. Music can permeate an environment and penetrate the listener; a piece of visual art can stop people in their tracks and jar them into seeing something differently; a play can evoke a range of emotions, causing audience members to weep and laugh. Clearly not all art, or even most art, affects people in these ways; however various arts have the capability of doing so. Even when a particular art piece falls below these lofty goals, it may still communicate an important story or range of meanings, and do so in an aesthetically interesting way. Given the various aesthetic qualities of art forms, it is not surprising that many people take pleasure in the beauty of the arts and their power to transform, alter mood or outlook, and bring depth to life. The arts as a representational form therefore accomplish two important things formerly absent from social research reports.

First, the appeal of the arts extends beyond academia, as does the ability for a novice to enter into the story being told (as Billy Collins suggests good poetry does). The turn toward artistic forms of representation brings social research to broader audiences, mitigating some of the educational and social class biases that have traditionally dictated the beneficiaries of academic scholarship. Although the goal of expanding the recipients of social research has yet to be met because most arts-based researchers still publish their work in specialized academic journals or present their work to limited audiences at conferences and the like, the potential is there in a way that is not the case with traditional jargon-laden social research reports and articles.

Second, the arts have the capability to evoke emotions, promote reflection, and transform the way that people think. The move toward artistic forms of representation in particular is entwined with the surge in social justice research within and across the disciplines. Many scholars using arts-based practices are doing so with the intent of increasing a critical consciousness, promoting reflection, building empathetic connections, forming coalitions, challenging stereotypes, and fostering social action.

Research conducted or presented via arts-based methods retains a transformational capability because of the oppositional potential of art as a medium. Historically, various art genres have been used as sites of resistance to social oppression. Grassroots movements, activist-artists, and many other individuals have drawn on the arts in social protest and resistance both publicly and privately. The resistive potential of art is now being harnessed by social researchers increasingly committed to dismantling stereotypes, accessing the voices of marginalized groups, and engaging in research that propels social change.

As new theoretical and epistemological perspectives, particularly those grounded in social justice politics, have emerged, a need for methodological innovation has also developed. The turn to the arts has been natural for some qualitative researchers because they view artistic inquiry as an extension of what qualitative researchers already do. In this regard, as noted throughout this volume, there is a congruency between the skills needed to conduct qualitative research and those that guide artistic practice. In summary, both practices can be conceived of as *crafts* aiming to shed light on some aspect of the social world and requiring that the researcher possess flexibility, creativity, intuition, storytelling proficiency, analytical ability, and openness. In addition to accessing and (re)presenting subjugated voices these methods are well suited to projects in which the researcher is after multiple meanings. In contrast to positivist research that limits the set of meanings that can emerge from a research project, arts-based practices lend themselves to multiplicity.

Figure 8.1 distinguishes some of the main features of quantitative research, traditional qualitative research, and arts-based research methods. This figure reveals several phenomena. First, arts-based practices are an extension of more conventional qualitative research while they also constitute a departure and ultimately an expansion of the qualitative paradigm. In this regard, arts-based practices can help qualitative

Quantitative	Traditional Qualitative	Arts-Based
Numbers	Words	Stories, images, sounds, scenes, sensory
Measurement	Meaning	Evocation
Tabulating	Writing	Re(presenting)
Value-neutral	Value-laden	Political, consciousness-raising, emancipation
Reliability	Process	Authenticity
Validity	Interpretation	Truthfulness
Prove/convince	Persuade	Compel
Disciplinary	Interdisciplinary	Transdisciplinary

FIGURE 8.1. Main tenets of quantitative, qualitative, and ABR approaches.

researchers facilitate their research goals, in ways not possible with traditional approaches. Moreover, these methods as a genre of the qualitative paradigm clearly move the paradigm forward. Specifically, the main features of these methods build on interpretive and critical perspectives while taking corresponding practices further than traditional approaches allow.

Second, arts-based practices require a different skill set on the part of the researcher than quantitative methods do. In this vein, the practice of arts-based methods may encourage traditional qualitative practitioners to further develop their research skills.

Third, building on the idea of going further with qualitative research skills, it is fair to say that arts-based practices are moving from interdisciplinary to transdisciplinary. In other words, former disciplinary boundaries are disrupted within the expanded qualitative paradigm—making way for integrated cross-disciplinary practices and emergent practices that are not "housed" in any one disciplinary context. This is another way in which these practices push the borders of existing research paradigms.

Finally, this figure indicates that the goals of arts-based practices— the *intention* within a given research project—differs from quantitative and traditional qualitative research purposes. Therefore, knowledge constructed with arts-based practices needs to be assessed on its own terms. Researchers working with this new breed of methods have been developing criteria for trustworthiness, authenticity, and validity, and it is important that broader scientific standards are adapted according to their findings so that the research community is not forced to compare apples and oranges. As noted throughout this book, appropriate evaluative standards may focus on vigor instead of the positivist-based rigor. Moreover, although new theoretical and methodological innovations are always met with scrutiny, and perhaps even fear, it is important to bear in mind that sometimes researchers are so careful to be "sterile" in their attempts to meet established scientific criteria and mitigate possible critique that they ironically end up *muddying up* the truths to be found in their work. In other words, reliance on the concepts of reliability and validity does not ensure that work will have any significance for the research community or the public.

We may also need to develop a new kind of practice-based language to explain and facilitate these new transdisciplinary research practices, including evaluative procedures. As qualitative research ushered in new terms appropriate with research practices, the new kind of knowledge-building occurring in arts-based traditions may also require a new way of talking about research. Many of the authors noted throughout this book are thinking in terms of *new research structures*. The research community needs to consider that knowledge can be developed and formed in new shapes linked to new ways of seeing. These new shapes are at times a sonic architecture or portraiture or many other forms. Using the language, practices, and forms of the arts allows us to think and therefore see in new ways.

As with all research projects, methods should be selected because they fit well with the research objectives. In other words, how well can this method or set of methods help answer the research question? What can this method access that would not be possible with other methods? What does this method fail to get at? Research objectives and the corresponding research design need to click. By *clicking together*, I mean to suggest that research methods should be selected and adapted to meet particular research questions that are embedded within a framework of epistemological assumptions and theoretical commitments. The arts-based practices reviewed in this book all try to achieve a harmony between research question, design, and final representation. Therefore, an arts-based approach may be appropriate when a traditional method does not fully address the research question or prevents a question from being formulated in accord with the intent of the researcher.

Moreover, an arts-based approach to research may constitute one phase of the project. For example, data collected and analyzed via conventional methods may later be represented via an artistic form in order to impart the particular kinds of meaning the researcher deems important and/or as a means of reaching a wider audience. Alternatively, data collected via traditional methods may be analyzed and interpreted with an arts-based practice. For example, interview of focus-group data may be analyzed using music as a model, allowing the data to be coded for timbre, dynamics, polyphony, and so on.

An arts-based practice may also serve as one method in a multimethod research project. In this case, the arts-based practice and traditional method(s) ideally inform each other, constituting an *integrated approach* to the methodology. For example, as noted in Chapter 6, Carol Picard combined traditional qualitative interviews, creative movement, and follow-up interviews and taped movement viewing in order to raise self-awareness and thus more fully access narratives about women's midlife experiences. The components of her research all spoke to each other. In this way, the multiple methods did not produce "more" data in the conventional sense, but rather each method shaped the data *as a whole*, adding depth, dimension, texture, and producing more openings through which the researcher and participant could enter to co-create meaning. This is the core of an integrated approach to research.

Arts-Based Research Practices

The methods practices reviewed in this book include narrative analysis, poetry, music, performance, dance and movement, and visual art. The techniques within these genres are all useful strategies for accessing silenced perspectives, evoking emotional responses, provoking dialogue, promoting awareness, and cultivating an increased social consciousness. The methods are not interchangeable, however, and each adapted art form features particular methodological strengths while requiring an understanding of the discipline from which it emerged. Here I briefly review some key aspects of how these various art forms can be refashioned as research practices and what they are most suited to reveal.

Narrative Analysis

Narrative has long held a central role in social research, with the sharing of stories being a primary qualitative research practice enabled by various methods. Likewise, writing has always been an integral component of social research. In both quantitative and qualitative research, results are typically reported or explained in textual form, making writing the major communicative device of scientific research. Qualitative researchers generally use writing during all phases of the research endeavor. For example, ethnographers systematically write down their observations as well as various kinds of memo notes in which they also document their impressions. Content analysts, whether deductive or inductive, draw themes and codes out of the data, all of which is expressed in written form. Moreover, qualitative data yielded from many methods are frequently communicated in narrative form. For example, oral history and in-depth interview data are often written as a linear, episodic, or thematic stories. In these ways and others, writing, and even the story format more specifically, are inseparable components of the research process.

In recent decades there has been a move within the qualitative paradigm to account for the place of the researcher within the text. In this regard, there has been a rise in the explicit use of autobiographical data (evidenced, for example, by autoethnography). The attention now paid to the place of the researcher within the text stems from concerns regarding voice and disclosure as well as increased theoretical commitments to how power operates via the representation of research findings (a primary concern raised by postmodern theory). The heightened awareness of power in the writing process is also linked to rises in reflexivity in both theory and practice. Douglas Macbeth defines *reflexivity* as "a deconstructive exercise for locating the intersections of author, other, text, and world, and for penetrating the representational exercise itself" (2002, p. 35). Our understanding of reflexivity has expanded from a focus on the ways that biography shapes research to include a critical disruption of the traditional writing and representation process. The growth in narrative research is interlinked with the elaborated use of autobiographical data and practices in reflexivity.

In addition, the short story format, fiction, experimental writing forms, and other literary devices have been adapted in order to most vibrantly communicate data from autoethnographic research as well as data collected via more traditional qualitative methods. The merging of ethnographic data, autobiographical data, and fiction allows researchers to communicate the textured nature of social life while illuminating the link between individual experience and the macro context in which that experience occurs. In this regard, the literature on metaphor within qualitative research has also expanded with metaphors being used to solve problems, assist interpretive practices, and link the micro and macro levels of social analysis during the writing-up of research results (see Dexter & LaMagdeleine, 2002; Moring, 2001; Todd & Harrison, 2008).

Poetry

Poetry is a literary form that relies on words, sound, and space—all carefully crafted in order to evoke meaning(s). A unique writing form, poetry can reveal aspects of human life that are obscured by traditional prose. In this regard, Eisner writes, "Poetry was invented to say what words can never say. Poetry transcends the limits of language and evokes what cannot be articulated" (1997, p. 5). Poetry can interrupt traditional ways of knowing and steer us in new directions. The crafting of research poems involves a drastic reduction in data, and the resulting poem represents a heightened glimpse into some aspect of social life. In this sense, poems can represent the *essence* of a topic in a vivid, sensory scene. As autoethnography and other methods of self-study are increasing, many researchers are also finding poetry to be an appropriate representational form.

Music

Music is a penetrating force in social life, able to enter a person's body in a profound and immediate way. Anthropologists have been at the forefront of interrogating how music serves as a window into cultural and political aspects of social life, including the productive role of culture (making music a constituent part of social life and not merely an addendum to it). Furthermore, anthropologists have also created cross-disciplinary methods working directly with the tenets of musicology to create hybrid methods like ethnomusicology. With regard to the continuum of arts-based research practices, music represents a departure from word-based forms into a performance-based arena. Although music has its own language for notation purposes, it comes into being via performance, and so music-based research methodologies typically focus on performed music. Moreover, the performance of music, as well as the experience of listening to it, merges the mind and body; making music and listening to it necessarily embodied experiences.

Methodologically, the most recent innovations involve using music as a model for qualitative research. Developing hearing skills, particularly in the context of a visual world, can assist researchers in attaining the listening skill set that is critical to successful ethnographic or interview research. In addition, attention to the various components of music—form, rhythm, dynamics, timbre, polyphony, melody—can call our attention to often veiled dimensions of our data as well as our interpretive and writing process. In this way, music can be used as a model for the analysis and interpretation of interview data, as well as the writing/representation of research findings. Within this framework new methods, such as Jenoure's (2002) musical portraiture method, are now developing. These sonic-based research practices are opening up a whole new language for interpreting and writing up or presenting qualitative data.

Performance Studies

Performance is a mode of storytelling involving an immediate transfer between the actors and audience. During this exchange, meaning is imparted, negotiated, and multiplied. In social research, performance can be used both as a tool of investigation and a form of representation. A methodological genre in its own right, performance-based methods are diverse and are used for many different purposes. Performance and theater can be used as a pedagogical tool, empowerment tool, a means of personal growth, or a healing tool. In the context of social research, performance can be used for consciousness-raising, discovery, subversion, and community-building.

Constructing a research performance script differs from the traditional writing up of qualitative data. Both processes involve a reduction of data, crafting, and may involve a "restorying," but the writing of a performance script explicitly involves reducing the data to the most dramatic parts. Moreover, even when the data being used comes from interview research and the like, the interviewees still need to be transformed into "characters." The process of characterization involves many choices. For example, how many characters will the script require? Will composite characters be created? What will the characterization process entail? How will dialogue and monologue be created? What methods will be used to represent discordant data? What role will the researcher have in the script? How will participants' privacy be safeguarded?

Unlike a written text, an ethnodramatic script is an unfolding narrative with multimedium components. Researchers must consider the visual aspects of the performance, such as costuming, scenery, and lighting, as well as the plot, storyline, and overall play structure. Public performances of research data increase awareness of the issues under scrutiny to ensure high standards of participant well-being, with the added issue of protecting audience well-being.

Dance and Movement

Dance is an embodied activity and an abstract art form that exists in the moment. As an expressive therapy like music, dance and movement can be used to build positive self-esteem and heal physical ailments. Beyond its utility as a therapeutic tool, dance can be adapted as a research method (for data collection or representation) and is particularly well suited to projects focused on discovery and exploration. Systematic methods of studying movement, such as LMA, provide rigorous procedures for investigating a fluid art form. Dance and movement are also useful in multimethod research in which they can add dimensionality to data garnered in more conventional ways, such as interview. In this regard, dance can be employed as a part of an integrated approach where there is a congruency between the research purpose and method. Finally, dance is an alternative representational form that allows data to be communicated to audiences in ways that maximize the *tonality* of lived experience. Experimental forms like dance are now present at conferences in education and sociology, indicating that there are professional forums outside of the arts in which this representational method can be tested.

The Visual Arts

Historically, many disciplines have had a visual art or image component. As noted in the last chapter, visual anthropology gave rise to photography as a research tool, which has been adapted in many ways. Nowadays visual sociology is also a recognized specialization. The expansion of the visual arts into interdisciplinary and transdisciplinary methodological innovations is, however, relatively new.

Visual images are a powerful communicative tool with the potential to help us see things in new ways. Therefore, researchers are using visual imagery as a part of data analysis as well as a medium to represent data, often with the intent of confronting and challenging stereotypes and the prevailing ideology that normalizes them. In this vein, bell hooks (1995) explains that people can see familiar things in visual art for the purpose of identification (and at times juxtaposed with images that jar us into seeing something differently), and that art can also defamiliarize, forcing people to see old ideas in new ways (such as racist or sexist historical images presented in a new context). Visual art challenges viewers in an immediate and visceral way while remaining open to a multiplicity of meanings. Many research methods involve the use of preexisting art. Participatory arts-based methods call on research participants to create art as data, whereas other methods, such as collage, call on the researcher to juxtapose found images in intentional ways that impart a set of meanings. A host of methods and techniques are available for qualitative researchers interested in using visual art. Moreover, traditional qualitative methods of coding visual imagery can be adapted to suit many arts-based projects. In addition, with the advent of the Internet, digital photography, and other technological advances, visual arts-based practices are only increasing, as is the need for widespread discussion of the ethical implications of some of these newer technology-based practices.

Exploding Myths and Building Coalitions: Crossing the Art and Science Divide

The scholar seeks, the artist finds.
—ANDRE GIDE

Art is mysterious. Science is straightforward. Art promotes thought through its reliance on metaphor, symbolism, and imagination. Science offers "facts" and "truth" through its reliance on numbers, words, and objectivity.

These kinds of polarizing and one-dimensional views of artistic practice and scientific inquiry have guided the building of paradigmatic borders within which artistic inquiry and social inquiry have been artificially separated. However, a serious interrogation of qualitative practice from *within the qualitative paradigm* has resulted in landscape-changing advances in theoretical and methodological work.

Moreover, the dismantling of the dichotomies that guide positivist research, including the rational–emotional, subject–object, and concrete–abstract, as reviewed in Chapter 1, have ultimately led to the discovery and interrogation of additional dualistic models that have underscored social scientific research practice while remaining invisible and thus beyond discourse. These dichotomies are: science–art and fact–fiction. Arts-based research practices call our attention to the polarizing notions that distinguish art and science from each other in ways that have prevented the kinds of cross-breeding that might advance conversations about the human condition and our study of it. For example, art–science innovations call our attention to the power of art to interrogate and communicate and the many ways that metaphor, symbolism, and imagination already guide qualitative "scientific" practice, although within the shadows. In these ways and others, arts-based innovations and the public scrutiny of them by various professional communities allow the scientific community to problematize the polarization of fact and fiction—an artificial dualism that legitimizes some ways of knowing over others and may contribute to the replication of dominant power relations.

The fusion of tools from the arts with scientific methods has created the methodological innovation necessary to more fully address the complex realities that constitute social life. With this said, arts-based practices have a long way to go with respect to professional legitimacy and technical efficiency. This genre is exciting in part because these methods have not reached their potential. Continued research with and about these practices is necessary in order to help researchers get the most out of their use.

Pragmatically, in order for the best researchers to be able to work with these methods as appropriate to their research projects, the institutional context in which research occurs needs to change. For instance, arts-based practices cannot be relegated to the status of second- or third-tier methods. These methods cannot be categorized as "experimental," which serves to undermine and marginalize these practices. In order to advance our understanding of these practices and their potential to add to our knowledge, conference, publication, and funding opportunities need to be available for researchers using these less-conventional methods. As Sharlene Hesse-Biber and I (2006) wrote about in our book on emergent methods, a "funding gap," often coupled with the pressure to publish in recognized peer-reviewed forums, prevents researchers from engaging in cutting-edge methodology. As academia has become more interdisciplinary, these material and structural barriers should be adjusted to make way for methodological hybrids like those reviewed in this volume. As evidenced by the suggested journals and websites listed at the end of each chapter in this book, opportunities to work with these methods and still meet professional benchmarks of publication and the like are increasingly available. For the time being, researchers beginning to work with these methodological practices may meet some resistance by the established scientific community. Cubist painter Georges Braque once famously noted: "Art upsets, science reassure" (Fitzhenry, 1993, p. 51) It may help to bear this in mind when bumping up against institutional and pragmatic barriers.

While individual researchers may not feel empowered to change the institutional landscape in which research occurs, they can take measures to elevate the quality of their arts-based research, the cumulative impact of which may change the status of these practices. Here I propose two related suggestions: greater attention to aesthetics and the building of cross-disciplinary research partnerships.

Although experimenting with new forms is an important part of professional growth, researchers intending to represent their data with arts-based methods must learn the rules of the discipline they are adapting in order to strengthen their representation. In particular, the aesthetic qualities that help to define the arts cannot be lost in translation. Put differently, the final representation should be able to stand on its own as a piece of art while simultaneously communicating information. This does not mean that community-produced art and the like must be "arresting" in order to be worthwhile, but rather that as novices are brought into the artistic enterprise considerations should be made for enhancing the quality of the art. In order to accomplish this difficult task, bridges need to be built between artists and social science researchers. Through these partnerships and coalitions each can assist the other as he or she crosses disciplinary boundaries. As hands-on research and teaching networks are created, so too will methods and art fuse to create new avenues for social research.

REFERENCES

Dexter, S., & LaMagdeleine, D. R. (2002). Dominance theater, slam-a-thon, and cargo cults: Three illustrations of how using conceptual metaphors in qualitative research works. *Qualitative Inquiry, 8*(3), 362–380.

Eisner, E. W. (1997). The promise and perils of alternative forms of data representation. *Educational Researcher, 26*(6), 4–10.

Fitzhenry, R. I. (Ed.). (1993). *The Harper book of quotations* (3rd ed.). New York: HarperPerennial.

Hesse-Biber, S. N., & Leavy, P. (2006). *Emergent methods in social research.* Thousand Oaks, CA: Sage.

hooks, b. (1995). *Art on my mind: Visual politics.* New York: The New Press.

Jenoure, T. (2002). Sweeping the temple: A performance collage. In C. Bagley & M. B. Cancienne (Eds.), *Dancing the data* (pp. 73–89). New York: Peter Lang.

Macbeth, D. (2001). On "reflexivity" in qualitative research: Two readings, and a third. *Qualitative Inquiry, 7*(1), 35–68.

Moring, I. (2001). Detecting fictional problem solvers in time and space: Metaphors guiding qualitative analysis and interpretation. *Qualitative Inquiry, 7*(3), 346–369.

Pollock, D. (2006). Performance trouble. In D. S. Madison & J. Hamera (Eds.), *The Sage handbook of performance studies* (pp. 1–8). Thousand Oaks, CA: Sage.

Todd, Z., & Harrison, S. J. (2008). Metaphorical analysis. In S. Hesse-Biber & P. Leavy (Eds.), *Handbook of emergent methods* (pp. 479–494). New York: Guilford Press.

Author Index

Subject Index

273

About the Author

Patricia Leavy, PhD, is Associate Professor of Sociology, Chairperson of the Sociology and Criminology Department, and the Founding Director of the Gender Studies Program at Stonehill College in Easton, Massachusetts. She is the author of *Iconic Events: Media, Politics, and Power in Retelling History* (2007); coauthor of *Feminist Research Practice: A Primer* (2007) and *The Practice of Qualitative Research* (2006); and coeditor of *Approaches to Qualitative Research: A Reader on Theory and Practice* (2003), *Emergent Methods in Social Research* (2006), *Handbook of Emergent Methods* (2008), and *Hybrid Identities: Theoretical and Empirical Examinations* (2008). Dr. Leavy is regularly quoted in newspapers for her expertise in popular culture and gender and has appeared on CNN's *Glenn Beck Show* as well as *Lou Dobbs Tonight*.

Contributors

Mary Beth Cancienne, PhD, is Assistant Professor in the Department of Middle, Secondary, and Mathematics Education in the College of Education at James Madison University, Harrisonburg, Virginia. For more than 8 years she has taught creative movement in learning courses to K–12 inservice teachers. Dr. Cancienne's research interests and publications explore movement as a method for theorizing, researching, and teaching. She publishes journal articles in the area of arts-based research and is the coauthor of a book and CD-ROM titled *Dancing the Data* (2002).

Diane Conrad, PhD, is Associate Professor of Drama/Theatre Education in the Department of Secondary Education, University of Alberta, Edmonton, Alberta, Canada. Her research engages youth in applied theater processes combining critical pedagogy and participatory arts-based inquiry. Dr. Conrad's current award-winning research project is with incarcerated youth to investigate the contribution participatory drama can make to their education, to help avoid future negative outcomes of their behaviors. Recent publications include "Rethinking 'At-Risk' in Drama Education: Beyond Prescribed Roles" in *Research in Drama Education* and "Justice for Youth versus a Curriculum of Conformity in Schools and Prisons" in the *Journal of the Canadian Association for Curriculum Studies.*

Norma Daykin, PhD, is Director of the Arts and Health Research Programme within the Centre for Public Health Research at the University of the West of England, Bristol, United Kingdom. A sociologist with multidisciplinary interests, her current research includes investigation of the role of music in health care as well as examination of issues of aesthetics in relation to public policy. Dr. Daykin has extensive experience of research and publications focused on the social aspects of health, as well as on health care evaluation research. Her current projects include a 2-year Department of Health–funded evaluation of "Moving On," an arts and mental health initiative in Avon and the Wiltshire

Mental Health Partnership NHS Trust, and evaluation of the "ArtLift" project, a Gloucester-based initiative that offers participatory arts to patients within primary care settings. Dr. Daykin's research also encompasses user involvement, cancer care, health professions, employment issues, and gender. She played a key role in the recently completed national evaluation of the NHS Patient Advice and Liaison Service and in the 3-year project completed in 2003 evaluating and developing best practices in user involvement within Avon, Somerset, and Wiltshire Cancer Services.

Carolyn Jongeward, EdD, is a visual artist who also has a career in education and research. In 1995 she completed her doctorate at the Ontario Institute for Studies in Education, University of Toronto, specializing in adult education. Dr. Jongeward's dissertation, *Connecting with Creativity*, describes processes that occur when adults learn to value and develop their creativity. Her creative process is the subject of the book *Weaver of Worlds* (1990). Since 1997 Dr. Jongeward's research projects have focused on international development issues of women, culture, and livelihoods. She has written extensively about the efforts of community-based organizations in less-developed countries to enable women to produce and market fine textiles and other handmade objects.

Cynthia Cannon Poindexter, MSW, PhD, is Faculty Research Scholar at the Ravazzin Center for Social Work Research in Aging and Associate Professor at the Fordham University Graduate School of Social Service where she teaches HIV policy, HIV practice, and supervision. She has been a practitioner in the human services field for 26 years, 16 of those years in the HIV field. Dr. Poindexter's research includes HIV education, older HIV-affected caregivers, and HIV service provision.

Karen Scott-Hoy, DocPhDEd, has been involved in community development and adult education in Australia for the past two decades. The author of numerous papers and publications, she uses visual art, narrative, and auto-ethnography to interrogate her research topics and herself as a researcher, allowing multiperspectival reflection on the social phenomena. Dr. Scott-Hoy is currently associated with the Centre for Research in Education, Equity, and Work at the University of South Australia.

Celeste N. Snowber, PhD, is a dancer, writer, and educator, and an Associate Professor in the Faculty of Education at Simon Fraser University outside Vancouver, British Columbia, Canada. She has focused her work in the area of embodiment, spirituality, arts/dance education, and arts-based inquiry. Dr. Snowber has written numerous essays and poetry in journals and chapters in books in the areas of the arts, holistic education, and curriculum studies. She is author of *Embodied Prayer*, which is in its second edition and has been translated into Korean, and author of *In the Womb of God*. Dr. Snowber has published her poems in various journals and has created outdoor site-specific performances that include dance and poetry in sites near the ocean. She is presently finishing a volume of poetry and a book on sexuality and spirituality.

Maryjean Viano Crowe, PhD, uses materials in unique ways to create large-scale photographic tableaux, artist books, and mixed-media constructions, including clothing and light-box shrines. Her work was the subject of a feature article in *Popular Photography* in 1992 and is featured in numerous private and museum collections, including the Polaroid International Collection and the Bibliothèque Nationale in Paris. In 1995 Dr. Viano Crowe received a fellowship from the National Endowment for the Arts; in 1987 she received a Massachusetts Artists Foundation Fellowship, for which she was a three-time finalist. Her work is featured in several books, including *Photomontage: A Step-by-Step Guide to Building Pictures* (1997), *Altered Books* (2003), and *The Book of Alternative Photographic Processes* (2002). Her work most recently appears in *Mixed Media Collage* (2007).